The Methu

How the science of anti-aging can he.. ....uppier, longer and stronger

By James Lee

Note – This book was previously known as The Science of Longevity.

Important Disclaimer

The information provided in this book is designed to provide helpful information on the subjects discussed. This book is not meant to be used, nor should it be used, to diagnose or treat any medical condition. For diagnosis or treatment of any medical problem, consult your own physician. The publisher and author are not responsible for any specific health or allergy needs that may require medical supervision and are not liable for any damages or negative consequences from any treatment, action, application or preparation, to any person reading or following the information in this book. References are provided for informational purposes only and do not constitute endorsement of any websites or other sources.

Contents

Part 1 – Introduction and background

The human obsession with long life and immortality predates even the mythical *Fountain of Youth*, which was a mythical spring thought to bestow immortality on whomever drank from it or bathed in it. Spanish explorer Juan Ponce de León reputedly stumbled on what would become modern day Florida while searching for it in the 1600s. Even before this, the Fountain of Youth was referred to in the writings Herodotus some legends surrounding Alexander the Great. Likewise, the *Elixir of Life* mentioned in Chinese, Indian and European mythology reportedly confers similar benefits to whoever should be fortunate enough to drink it.

However, surely in mythology the undisputed king of long life must be Methuselah, who *reportedly* (and I use that term loosely) lived to the ripe old age of 969. Many scholars quite soberly reject this claim, saying that his actual age was either mistranslated (and was actually closer to 96.9 years old) or that the story is not meant to be taken literally. Taking a moment to imagine what it would be like to live to 969 is actually quite helpful because most people assume they would choose immortality if they had the choice. When you start to imagine each 50 year block, you realize why the finite human lifespan is actually a great gift. I can't imagine what Methuselah would have done to occupy himself for all those years besides woodworking and shooing teenagers off his lawn. *Matlock* didn't start showing on TV until the 1980s, well after Methuselah died, so it is hard to imagine how he spent his evenings.

In modern times, this same basic desire to live as long as possible has led to the science of anti-aging, which is dedicated to extending lifespan and making these additional years happy and productive. After all, it would be pointless to live until you were 150 if you spend those last 50 years in a wheelchair, with just a faint pulse signaling to loved-ones that you are indeed still alive.

When people think of anti-aging, they think of oxidative stress, antioxidants, expensive face creams and the like. However this is far too narrow a definition for anti-aging as I see it. I prefer to use the term life-extension, which is more descriptive of what it is I am looking to achieve with this book. Oh, and in the interests of disclosure, this book contains no secret tips on how to keep your skin looking its best – there are more than enough books on that already.

Life extension is not just about eating broccoli and lathering *Crème de la Mer* on your face each night. It's also about playing the odds. Each poor decision you make regarding your health accumulates. For example, imagine that you smoke a pack a day of cigarettes ever each, drink a six pack of beer each night, drink a liter of Coca Cola each day while you work, take cocaine on weekends with your buddies, ride a high-powered motorbike everywhere (sometimes without a helmet), go skydiving each weekend, surf in an area notorious for great white sharks, have a high-stress job, rarely eat fruit or vegetables and eat a diet based primarily around junk food.

How long do you think you will live? Each of your poor diet and lifestyle choices is like playing a game of Russian roulette. One day there will be a bullet in the chamber. So life extension is about a holistic plan that incrementally decreases your odds of dying by misadventure or developing a preventable disease. This is all about reducing risk, not about guaranteeing anything. Sometimes people can become fatalistic when they hear of the health fanatic that dropped dead at 40 with a heart attack. *If it can happen to that guy, why bother?*

There are always going to be exceptions and people with certain genetic issues that may predispose them to particular problems. However the fact remains that if you make good choices, take good care of yourself and follow some basic nutritional and supplemental principles, you will dramatically increase your odds of making it to 100 and beyond.

Some researchers have more ambitious targets, believing that we have a potential maximum life span of 150 years or more. Some even believe there is no theoretical maximum and if they crack the code we could live indefinitely.

Me personally, I would be comfortable with 100. I think that by the time I reach that age, I will be well and truly ready to throw in the towel and move on to whatever awaits me on the other side, if anything.

You are holding in your hand a guide to getting to whatever your personal target age may be. Firstly I want to give you some of the science that underpins the concept of aging and what we can do to work around some of the impediments to a long and healthy life. Then I will go through some of the practical steps you can take to get you where you want to go.

Originally, aging was viewed as the natural process of wear and tear your body goes through as it fights the *second law of thermodynamics*. The second law of thermodynamics refers to a range of universal concepts, including the fact that heat will transfer from warmer to cooler areas over time, leading to equal temperatures. This is why a glass of water left at room temperature will eventually move towards whatever the ambient temperature is (all other things being equal). However the second law of thermodynamics also states that compound, ordered bodies (anything with mass) in a closed system will gradually move towards disorder. This is often misconstrued to refer to processes such as the decay of a dead body or a piece of wood rotting in the ground. So originally, aging was viewed as your body moving inexorably towards disorder, and when it reached a particular tipping point (through damage or whatever mechanism), death would occur.

However the problem with all this "second law of thermodynamics" talk is that it wasn't actually correct. The aging of the human body has nothing to do with the second law because the human body isn't a closed system. Your body is constantly taking in energy and nutrients from your environment for metabolic functions and general repair – it doesn't operate in a vacuum.

Let me use an analogy – Say you are made of building blocks that look just like the blocks little babies use to build things, and next to you is an inexhaustible pile of replacement blocks. Each time one of your blocks breaks, you can just grab a new block and slide it into place just where the old, broken one had been. In this scenario, you would not be breaking the second law by continuing to exist in perpetuity.

Similarly, sometime in the 19th century, this idea that aging was an unavoidable consequence of the second law was discredited and abandoned. Well not entirely. The second law is to this day sometimes misappropriated in Creationist circles as a means to explain why evolution violates this fundamental principle of the universe, with *intelligent design* is the only logical explanation.

This is an exciting concept to ponder. Due to the fact that animals are constantly swapping energy and other "stuff" with their environment, there is no theoretical reason why humans or other animals could not achieve immortality. However, clearly when you think about it, immortality would, on balance be a terrible idea for just about every living creature on earth. Which is why biology appears to have put in place a range of self-destruct mechanisms designed to keep populations of animals young, strong and healthy. Unburdened by a large population of elderly specimens.

Despite the fact that this process is occurring essentially from birth (or some may say, from early adulthood when growing has stopped and decay starts to accelerate), aging generally becomes noticeable only from middle age as things start to malfunction and break. Another way to look at this is that your body undergoes constant repair and regeneration work throughout life. However, as you age, slowly your body starts struggling to keep up with this repair work. It is thought that certain types of cancers start in this way. Researchers believe that quite regularly, certain cells mutate and become potentially cancerous, however they are quickly eliminated by your immune system. As you age, these mutations increase, making it harder for your immune system to keep up and more likely that one of these mutant cells will be missed – leading to cancer.

However it is not purely environmental aging at work, but also a complex interaction between your genetics and your environment. In the past, people often referred to "nature versus nurture", which was basically referring to genes and environment. Was someone born that way or did something happen to them that triggered a certain illness or behavior? However nowadays as science has progressed, the buzz word has become epigenetics, which basically refers to your genes and how they can be turned on or off by your environment. Let me give the example of a smoker. Why is it that some people can smoke a pack a day for life and never get lung cancer while others are struck down in midlife, despite smoking the same amount of cigarettes? This is because a small minority of smokers have a particular genetic makeup that prevents them from developing lung cancer. I should point out an important point however – many smokers point to these rare outliers who don't get cancer as a reason why it doesn't matter whether you smoke or not. However this is a complete fallacy. Not only are these people exceedingly rare, this belief doesn't take epigenetics into account. You should never base your beliefs and decisions on the visible minority (they are the visible minority because most of the other long-term smokers are not particularly visible unless you are a *"Long Island medium"*)

So any scientific research aimed at extending the life span of humans must also look at genetics, not just environmental aging. As Danica Chen, UC Berkeley's assistant professor of Nutritional Science and Toxicology states *"A major goal of the aging field is to utilize knowledge of genetic regulation to treat age-related diseases."*

In a nutshell, irrespective of whether we are looking at genetics or environmental aging, anti-aging research is focused on slowing down, inhibiting or reversing the process of aging to increase the human life span.

There is also a philosophical debate in scientific fields as to whether the aging process should be viewed as a disease or a natural process. Harvard Medical School's David Sinclair says *"I don't see aging as a disease, but as a collection of quite predictable diseases caused by the deterioration of the body"*. In contrast, David Gems, Assistant Director of the Institute of Healthy Aging, believes that aging must be considered as a form of disease. However irrespective of the philosophy underpinning the science, the fact remains that all researchers are united in their ambition to both extend the human life span and make any extra years pleasant and disability free for as many people as possible. And coming out of this work over the past two decades has been some amazing advances in our understanding of the process of aging and potential ways in which these processes can be modulated.

Aging is a complicated process that includes a range of parameters health, cognitive function, and level of physical mobility. Who is actually older – the 80 year old who can run a marathon and write a novel or a 30 year old with type-2 diabetes that sits on the couch all day because of a bad back and muscle soreness? As part of this thinking we need to broaden our definition of anti-aging far beyond the concept of life-extension. I think a better target would be *"life-extension + life-optimization"*.

Despite this, some researchers believe that by targeting one, you naturally target the other. The latest issue of the *Public Policy & Aging Report (PP&AR)*, titled *The Longevity Dividend:*

Geroscience Meets Geropolitics, states that the best way to achieve improved longevity and quality of life is by targeting the slowing down of the process of biological aging rather than targeting the individual diseases separately.

Life expectancy and life span

It is when we look at life expectancy rather than life span that we can see why the definition of anti-aging needs to be expanded away from narrow areas of focus such as oxidative stress. In 2002, scientists pointed out that life expectancy is has been on a continuous upward trend for the past 160 years, with life expectancy increasing by a quarter of a year annually. This average life-expectancy (defined as the average number of years a person will live) - has increased from 46 years at the start of the 20th century to 65 years today. However, the irrefutable fact during the same period is that the maximum potential lifespan hasn't changed in that whole time. Not only does this call into question our ability to extend this maximum lifespan (at the time of writing the oldest person to have lived – and been verified – so Methuselah doesn't count - was France's Jeanne Calment, who lived to 122), but also points to the important point I made earlier – life-expectancy is determined by a range of factors, not just chronological aging. In the last hundred years or so, the biggest driver of increased life expectancy by far has been our ability to treat infectious diseases which were previously often fatal. Some awful diseases (such as smallpox), have been virtually wiped off the planet. When you stop to ponder this you realize that any effort to extend your own personal lifespan to 100 and beyond (with your physical health and faculties intact) must tackle the problem from multiple angles, not just slowing down chronological aging.

So while we will continue to see increases in life expectancy (particularly in the area of cancer research and improvements in our understanding of heart disease), until a truly major breakthrough is made, any improvements on our maximum life span will only ever be incremental. Put another way, as lifestyle and medical care continues to improve, more people with "longevity-friendly" genes will survive long enough to seriously challenge Jeanne Calment's record.

However don't give up hope. After all, at various times over the past few decades certain scientists have claimed that we would not see any more improvements in life expectancy. Yet we continue to see improvements each year, little by little. So while I can't see anything on the near horizon that would extend life span much beyond current levels, I could be proven wrong with a single major discovery or development.

Nevertheless, the focus of this book will be on increasing your own personal life expectancy, not your maximum life span. If someone promises to help you live to 130, don't hand over any money!

In terms of life expectancy, Japan remains the clear front-runner among major countries with a large enough sample size (Smaller locations such as - Monaco with an average life expectancy of 89.63 years and Macau with 84.46 years don't have a big enough sample size to draw sweeping conclusions). Japan has an impressive life expectancy of 84.19 years for men and women combined. In fact, in Japan alone there are more than 50,000 centenarians (those aged 100 years and above). This contrasts with countries like Chad, which have a disappointingly low life expectancy of 49.07 years. Curiously, not far from Chad, an Ethiopian farmer by the name of Dhaqabo Ebba has claimed to be over 160 years old. Ebba, who is, unsurprisingly, retired, has apparently lived through and witnessed a *"transfer of power among all of the five Gadaa Oromo political parties in four rotations"*, which would put his age at over 160. As he doesn't possess a birth certificate, scientists are currently working on verifying his age by other means. If his age is confirmed as being 160 years old, I will start getting my knife and fork, along with various condiments ready to consume my own hat.

Increases in life expectancy are now even capturing the attention of mainstream press, as evidenced by this article in the UK's *Guardian Newspaper* which said *""Every minute that you spend reading this article, the average life expectancy in Britain will rise by 12 seconds. By the time you finish reading, your life expectancy will have gone up by six minutes. This time tomorrow, it will have increased by almost five hours. The reason is clear: rapid advances in medicine and biology have been one of the biggest achievements of the past century and we are all living longer. Where anyone reaching the age of 60 was considered to be near death's door at the turn of the 20th century, it is barely old enough for retirement at the turn of the 21st century."* [14]

So, if the science is advancing so impressively, the next question must logically be – *What causes biological aging?*

Why and how do we age?

There are a massive number of theories on why and how we age. Many of these are not "either or" theories either, with their being a strong likelihood that the answer turns out to be a combination of factors. For example, it is highly likely that telomere shortening plays a role, along with oxidative stress also. However, broadly speaking, we can break the theories into two main groups –

1. "Programmed senescence" style theories – These theories say that we have an upper limit to our life span that is built into our genetics

2. "Damage" theories – These theories say that aging is caused by a range of changes caused by environmental damage. This damage can be "wear and tear" style damage or damage from genetic mutation caused by faulty repair processes.

According to programmed senescence style theories, aging is driven by an innate internal clock that is controlled by gene expression. Usually this internal clock is represented by telomeres, which sit at the end of chromosomes. Telomeres have been found to gradually shorten as an animal ages and this has been used as an example of how we have an internal process driving the aging process. However even this theory gets complicated due to the fact that many scientists believe that oxidative stress accelerates the process of telomere shortening.

Under these types of theories, any advances in longevity will require some form of modulation of this internal clock by, for example, slowing down telomere shortening somehow.

Under damage-style theories, it is believed that aging is caused by a range of processes which damage an organism. The organism either can't keep up its internal repair work or the repair work is faulty, leading to genetic mutations such as cancer. Two of the most commonly mentioned drivers of environmental aging are oxidative stress and inflammation. However there are a multitude of similar theories which could also be involved to some extent. For example, there is a theory linking life span with basal metabolic rate that proposes an inverse relationship between an animal's metabolic rate and how long it can possibly live for. So, under this theory, elephants would live a long time and hummingbirds much less so. This is probably one of the oldest theories as to why we age, being first proposed more than a century ago.

Now, before we move on to exactly *how* to slow down the aging process, let's familiarize ourselves with some of the core concepts and theories of aging in detail.

Senescence

At the cellular level, senescence refers to the point at which a cell ceases to divide. Based on experiments *in vitro* (in a test tube essentially), cells appear to have around 50 divisions before they become senescent and no longer divide. This upper limit to the number of divisions is known as the *Hayflick limit*. These senescent cells then just hang around, continuing to do their job until they are destroyed by other events (think of it as dying of natural causes). It is believed that these senescent cells hold one of the key clues to the aging process. In certain animal tests, removing senescent cells led to various improvements in age related conditions.

However, at various points during a cell's period of dividing (before reaching the *Hayflick limit*), certain external shocks or sudden damage can trigger a process known as apoptosis – programmed cell death. When a cell is damaged, attempts are made to repair the cell so it can continue to function. However in certain cases where the body decides that the damage is too great, it will trigger apoptosis and exterminate the cell.

The concept of senescence and apoptosis is central to any theory of aging because it touches on one of the great paradoxes of aging. You have probably read about apoptosis and senescence and thought - *Great! So why don't we just turn off this programmed cell death, allowing us to become immortal?* Well, there is one big problem – cancer. This is exactly what happens when apoptosis is switched off. At the cellular level, cancer begins when a cell suddenly decides that it won't commit cellular suicide and decides that rapid division instead is more its scene. This happens quite regularly however usually these cells are immediately identified and dealt with swiftly and without mercy. However, when the immune system is compromised or overloaded with these cells, that's when cancer has the chance to grow and spread.

This is why any tinkering with senescence and apoptosis needs to be done with extreme caution to ensure that cancer isn't the end result. Where this research gets truly interesting is in the studies of animals that do not appear to experience measurable senescence and do not appear to get cancer. The humble lobster is one example of this. Immortality or served on a plate with *mornay* sauce – there's no middle ground.

The equal and opposite of cancer is an accelerated aging disease such as *progeria*, where young children have tragically aged at such a dramatic rate that they look like elderly people. Any study of aging and related cancers could benefit from a deeper understanding of what drives these kinds of accelerated aging diseases.

A possible mechanism by which to clear out senescent cells and other cellular waste to slow down the aging process could be to optimize the natural process of *autophagy*. Autophagy is a process that keeps everything humming along nicely at the cellular level, preventing further damage that could come from harmful debris left floating around.

Not surprisingly, scientists have found that modulating the process of autophagy appears to trigger an anti-aging effect. The most promising example of this is in the area of caloric restriction for life extension. As of today, caloric restriction is arguably the single most potent and measurable life-extending technique we have at our disposal. A few years ago scientists noticed that you could dramatically increase the life span of various animals and organisms by restricting calorie consumption by a large proportion. This has also been validated in humans, where caloric restriction leads to improvements in a range of biomarkers for the aging process. As you could imagine, this is a tough sell for the general public. Most people surveyed usually indicate they would rather live a shorter life than spend the rest of their life eating celery. That includes me.

The other "great hope" of anti-aging supplements – resveratrol, was also found to exert its anti-aging effects via increased autophagy. Resveratrol is the substance extracted from grape skin (or *Japanese knotweed*) which is purported to slow down the aging process. When resveratrol was given to rodents who had their autophagy-related abilities disabled, it failed to give any anti-aging benefits. This appears to indicate that resveratrol perhaps confers some of its benefits via an ability to positively modulate your body's autophagy processes.

Scientists from Sanford-Burnham Medical Research Institute have found a substance that appears to play an important role in autophagy. It is a *transcription factor* (a protein that controls the movement of genetic information from DNA to mRNA) known as *HLH30*. This compound is the first identified transcription factor that is believed to be important in the longevity of *Caenorhabditis elegans* (a type of nematode roundworm) strains. A similar transcription factor, called *TFEB* has been shown to modulated autophagy in mice. Of particular interest is the role that TFEB plays in *Huntington' disease* – possibly the most severe of all genetically-modulated neurodegenerative disorders. Scientists are now studying ways to possibly increase expression of TFEB and reduce the neurotoxicity associated with Huntington's. Again, it appears as if caloric restriction increases expression of TFEB – perhaps pointing to another mechanism driving the anti-aging effect of restricting calories.

Telomere shortening

As mentioned earlier, telomeres sit at the end of chromosomes, gradually shortening after successive replications. Telomeres are often referred to using the rather accurate analogy of the piece of plastic that sits at the end of your shoelaces. Like these plastic caps, telomeres sit at the end of chromosomes, preventing them from "fraying", so to speak. However a more relevant analogy in the case of aging would be a bomb fuse. Telomeres, like a bomb fuse, can shorten to a point before – BOOM! – the cell self-destructs. Sorry, however this bomb analogy is about as exciting as cellular biology gets for some people. If you would permit me a third analogy, the function of telomeres is to act as a kind of fender for the chromosome. The telomere can take all the hits, slowly shortening, while protecting all the valuable DNA stored in the chromosome.

One of the reasons why telomeres shorten as the cell ages is that gradually levels of telomerase decrease. Telomerase adds length to the base of the telomere, slowing down the rate at which it shortens. The activity of telomerase is largely controlled by genes, so in 2010, Harvard researchers investigated the extent to which modulating the telomerase genes could have a beneficial effect on mice. *Jaskelioff et al* indeed found that by reactivating the telomerase activity, they were able to reverse a range of typical biomarkers of aging.

Free-radical theory

By far the most prominent theory on aging is known as the free-radical theory, and states that we gradually accumulate cellular damage caused by free radicals or *reactive oxygen species* (ROS). A free radical is any atom or molecule with an unpaired electron, whereas ROS are a type of free radical specific to oxygen molecules. Free radical damage is typically attributed to superoxide, hydrogen peroxide or peroxynitrite.

Normally electrons exist in pairs and are considered stable. In the case of a free radical with only a single electron, when it meets another molecule it will attempt to steal an electron from that molecule turning it also into a free radical. This can set off a chain reaction which leads to extensive damage at the cellular level through processes such as DNA cross-linking, which have been shown to potentially lead to cancer.

This is where antioxidants come to the rescue. Antioxidants can donate an electron to the free radical molecule without themselves becoming a free radical. Vitamin C is a great example of this, which is why it was the first real mainstream antioxidant that was proposed to counteract the damaging effects of free radicals. More on the use of antioxidants to prevent and reverse free radical damage later.

Unfortunately, ROS have been shown to reliably increase with age. What isn't as clear is which direction the arrow of causation travels. Does aging naturally trigger increased ROS or do elevated ROS accelerate aging? The weight of theoretical and practical evidence points to the latter, however more work is still required.

Mitochondrial dysfunction

The *mitochondrial theory of aging* is actually a sub-set of the *free radical theory*, as the majority of mitochondrial damage is proposed to be caused by free radicals.

Mitochondria are often referred to as your "cellular power plants" as they are responsible for the production of energy at the cellular level. Mitochondria are located in the cytoplasm of each cell (the part of the cell located outside the nucleus but inside the cell wall) and produce the main source of energy for the cell – *adenosine triphosphate* (ATP).

As your mitochondria are so central to the production of the energy which drives many cellular processes, it is unsurprising that scientists have investigated the anti-aging effects of improving mitochondrial function. Indeed, elderly subjects are consistently found to have significant decreases in mitochondrial function compared to younger subject. Two of the supplements with the best research into their positive effects on the mitochondria are coenzyme Q10 (CoQ10 or *ubiquinol*) and D-ribose.

Coenzyme Q10 plays a crucial role in the process of creating ATP at the cellular level, so it is hypothesized that by increasing levels of Co-Q10 by supplementation, you can optimize mitochondrial function to some extent. Co-Q10 is not just at the stage of pure theory or wild speculation. It is now regularly recommended by cardiologists for patients taking statins to reduce cholesterol. Statins reduce the absorption of certain fat soluble nutrients such as vitamin D and Co-Q10 so it is believed that by supplementing with Co-Q10 you are giving some much needed assistance to muscle cells that need Co-Q10 to function properly. This is one of the reasons why statin therapy is often associated with muscle soreness or weakness, as your muscles need these vital fat soluble nutrients for functioning and repair.

One of the reasons why CoQ10 is a no brainer supplement is that is also appears to function as a potent antioxidant. This means that irrespective of whether you believe the *mitochondrial dysfunction* theory or the *free-radical theory*, CoQ10 covers all bases. One of the most notable aspects of oxidative damage by free-radicals is *lipid* (fat) *peroxidation*. This is one of the reasons why CoQ10 is often promoted as a heart healthy supplement – it potently inhibits the oxidation of LDL, the cholesterol transporter molecule implicated in heart disease. CoQ10 reduces this peroxidation by inhibiting the production of *lipid peroxyl radicals*. CoQ10 also recycles other antioxidants such as vitamin E.

Discrepancies in mitochondrial function between males and females may also give us clues as to why women live longer than men on average. Researchers from the Monash School of Biological Sciences and Lancaster University looked at the aging differences between male and female fruit flies *(Side note – if you are wondering why scientists often use fruit flies, it is because they share around 75% of the same genetics as humans and are significantly lower maintenance than rodents and other mammals. If fruit fly research generates positive findings, researchers can move on to mammals and then hopefully on to humans later)*. They found that mitochondrial mutations appear to drive the speed of aging in male fruit flies but to a lesser extent in females. However I should point out that this is confounded by other factors such as the fact that the female immune system appears to retain function later in life compared to males.

Evolutionary theory

Evolution sits at the very heart of this topic as it is the forces of evolution that are largely responsible for our apparently swift descent into mortality. This is largely due to a single, central concept – over countless years, humans have been self-selected for durability against any disease that strikes down someone before they have the opportunity to breed. *Mother Nature* doesn't care if you get cancer or heart disease in your 60s – you have already (in most cases) created progeny to carry your genes. Naturally there are exceptions (including childhood cancers such as leukemia), however in general, if your genetics carry a potential weakness that can strike you down before you reach child-rearing age, as cold and bleak as it sounds, your genetic line will soon die out.

However, if your genetic code holds a predisposition to prostate cancer or heart disease, it will continue to be passed on, as it doesn't impact your ability to pass on your genes.

A version of this idea was one of the very first theories ever proposed to account for the apparent mystery as to why we age. This idea was called *Medawar's Hypothesis* - named after Sir Peter Medawar, famous British zoologist and Nobel Prize winner from the University of London. Nowadays it is usually referred to as the *mutation accumulation theory of aging*. Medawar used the example of *Huntington's disease*, which typically won't strike down someone who carries the genetic predisposition until after they have created offspring. Put another way, over the course of evolution, animals accumulate a range of genetic mutations, however it is only the mutations that cause problems after child rearing age that remain. Any mutations that strike down children or adolescents will soon be weeded out. So, under this theory, aging is simply a range of genetic mutations which have been passed on throughout history.

While this theory is attractive in the sense that it at least hints at the notion that aging is not an inescapable fact of life, there are some problems with it. The most obvious of these is that we now know that gene expression is rather more precise than previously thought when Medawar originally proposed his idea. Genes are typically programmed to express in a particular part of the body and at a particular time in a person's life, so it would be unlikely that animals evolve with the genetic coding to mutate by design during the latter stages of life.

However probably the final nail in the coffin for Medawar's theory was when, as part of the advances in our ability to understand genomics, it was discovered that there are genes for aging and they are not mutations. Some of the genes for aging are closely interwoven with other genes and these genes are often shared by organisms from man all the way to fungi. So clearly spontaneous mutations in one species could not explain the process of aging.

The American evolutionary biologist George Williams, building on the initial work of

Medawar, then proposed the *antagonistic pleiotropy hypothesis*, which states that there is an evolutionary cost to every beneficial genetic trait. So when applied to aging it states that we pay the price later in life for everything that has made us a robust species earlier in life. More specifically, it was proposed that aging and senescence was the price we pay for increased fertility and the ability to breed earlier and in greater numbers. However the main problem with this theory as it has not been backed up by the results of any experimentation. If there was an inverse relationship between longevity and fertility, breeding an animal for increased longevity should result in decreased fertility. However, as an example, an experiment using fruit flies found that the specimens bred for longer life actually become more fertile, not less.

To take this concept one step further, many have argued that we are indeed set up like printer cartridges are for *planned obsolescence*. Like a printer cartridge only has so many pages in it before the manufacturer has built in a kind of self-destruct function to boost sales, animals including humans appear to have our own self-destruct built in. This is in the form of various aging processes and diseases that target the elderly. The evolutionary purpose for this is clear – the more a population of animals is burdened by older specimens as a proportion of the total population, the weaker the group is as a whole.

The last of the major evolutionary theories is the *disposable soma theory* (original proposed by the biologist Thomas Kirkwood), which proposes the idea that an organism will prioritize vital functions ahead of repair work, assuming finite resources (finite energy, nutrition etc.). This theory proposes that the number one priority for an organism is to reach reproductive age and this rush to maturity means that other processes such as repair work can be sacrificed. Slowly over time, these small sacrifices accumulate as the aging process.

On the surface this may seem like a plausible theory however there is one major deal-breaker in my opinion – caloric restriction. One of the least disputed ideas in the field of aging is that restricting calories extends the life of an organism. So, under the disposable soma theory, restricting calories should lead to accelerated aging, not decreased aging.

Inflammation and *advanced glycation end-products* (AGEs)

Inflammation is one of the buzz words in medicine today – and for good reason. Each new emerging study appears to implicate inflammation in a range of diseases from multiple sclerosis to heart disease. Not to mention the conditions which are primarily inflammatory themselves, such as rheumatoid arthritis or inflammatory bowel disease.

Heart disease is the number one killer of middle-aged and older people, so any talk of life extension or anti-aging must take into consideration the mechanisms that underpin heart disease.

A vocal minority of cardiologists have, for some time now, been pointing to the "war on cholesterol" and highlighting something odd. Why in modern times do our arteries appear to suddenly start accumulating cholesterol deposits? If your body is sending cholesterol to your arteries in an attempt to patch up damage, what is causing that damage? Cholesterol is being deposited there for a reason – it's no bad guy. It's just trying to do a job. So the question should be what is causing this damage?

Gradually medical consensus is slowly turning towards chronic arterial inflammation as being a potential culprit. Doctors have known for a long time that heart disease is associated with inflammation – this is why a common test they will often arrange (called a CRP, or *C-reactive protein* test) looks for signs of inflammation. While everyone used to believe that heart disease caused inflammation, now there is a new hypothesis that asks whether inflammation causes heart disease.

Where this gets truly interesting is where there is now a gradually emerging idea that heart disease is not caused by saturated animal fat, but by trans-fatty acids, Omega-6 rich vegetable oils and sugar. Nothing is proven conclusively either way but one powerful piece of evidence is that reducing levels of these three foods in your diet (and keeping saturated fat unchanged or even increased), usually reduces CRP levels.

Put simply, any program that aims to increase longevity must tackle systemic inflammation as a priority. Inflammation damages cells, and each time your body needs to repair damage there is a minute chance of a mutation that could lead to cancer. Inflammation is one of the factors I can say conclusively is involved in accelerated biological aging.

A recent Yale study published in the journal *Cell Metabolism* identified the *Nlrp3 inflammasome* as the trigger for many of the age-related problems that appear to be either triggered or influenced by inflammation. To put this another way, this study found that the general systemic inflammation which often increases with age isn't a natural consequence, but is turned on by the *Nlrp3 inflammasome*. Where this area of inquiry will get truly interesting is when we are able to prevent *Nlrp3* from doing its job, possibly preventing a range of inflammatory diseases that reduce life expectancy.

Indeed, initial mouse experiments have shown that by reducing the activity of *Nlrp3* the test subjects appeared to be protected from a range of age-related conditions such as dementia, bone loss and glucose intolerance.

Recently Zhang et al, from Albert Einstein College of Medicine found that at least some of the inflammatorily mediated aging we see appears to be related to inflammation in the hypothalamus. The hypothalamus is the part of your brain central to the control of autonomic functions and hormonal control. These researchers found that inflammation in the hypothalamus appeared to trigger a range of age-related health problems such as metabolic syndrome. This inflammation appeared to be controlled by NF-κB (nuclear factor kappa-light-chain-enhancer of activated B cells that regulates transcription of DNA). The researchers found that when they blocked the the NF-κB pathway in the hypothalamus, they saw a 20% increase in the longevity of test mice.

Inflammation has also been found to accelerate the production of *advanced glycation end products* (AGEs) which are usually formed when glucose binds with a protein, leading to cellular damage. The most common type of AGE that you would be familiar with is the browning of food, such as when something is caramelized. This is known as the *Maillard reaction* and involves the production of AGEs.

The damaging impact of AGEs in the body appears to be the subject of little debate. As Régis Moreau, Ph.D., a research associate at the Linus Pauling Institute states *"If we can prevent damage or remove existing damage caused by protein glycoxidation and maintain tissue integrity, we may be able to improve the health and vigor of the elderly"*. Stopping the formation of AGEs and repairing the ones that have already formed (or *cross-linked*) is the subject of considerable research at present.

However it should be pointed out that AGEs are not a completely separate aspect of anti-aging research and theory to oxidative stress. AGEs are seen as one of the main triggers for oxidative damage.

A 2010 study published in *Nutrients* also reached the conclusion that *"Although the data are not conclusive, the convergence of data from diverse experimental studies suggests an important role of AGEs in healthy aging, as well as chronic disease morbidity. Certainly the data are supportive that endogenous AGEs are associated with declining organ functioning. It appears that dietary AGEs may also be related...As of today, restriction of dietary intake of AGEs and exercise has been shown to safely reduce circulating AGEs, with further reduction in oxidative stress and inflammatory markers. More research is needed to support these findings and to incorporate these into recommendations for the elderly population."*

Interestingly, it is the concerns regarding the formation of AGEs that underpins some of the rationale for the raw food movement, which involves the consumption of uncooked, fresh food. Proponents believe that by avoiding cooked food, they are avoiding the unnecessary addition of AGEs to their diet. This is an interesting theory that deserves more study and it does indeed have logical grounding. However the problem I often observe with both raw food proponents and their vegan equivalents is that they often replace cooked meat with fruit and fruit juice high in fructose – one of the most powerful drivers of oxidative stress caused by AGEs.

Sirtuins

Another exciting field of inquiry at present is a type of protein called a *sirtuin*, which appears to play a role in controlling several aspects of longevity including apoptosis (programmed cell death), inflammation and cellular aging. In fact, if we look in closer detail at why resveratrol is a possible life-extender, it is linked to its ability to activate one of the sirtuins, *SIRT1*.

In a recent issue of *Science*, researchers have found that by targeting the enzyme *SIRT1 deacetylase*, they could achieve spectacular results such as increasing the life-span of rodents by more than 40%. Interestingly, this same pathway (activating SIRT1 deacetylase) appears to be one of the reasons why calorie restriction can work to increase life span.

So while scientists and biotech companies are working hard to develop therapies that specifically target SIRT1, until these new therapies become a reality your only option is resveratrol, caloric restriction or cardiovascular exercise. As if you didn't need another excuse to exercise more. You can now add *"increased SIRT1 deacetylase activity"* to exercise's long list of life-extending benefits. Don't forget to tell your gym buddies this in the locker room. You will be quite the popular one.

There is also considerable excitement regarding *SIRT3*, another sirtuin which is central to the process of mitochondrial function and the generation of stem cells. Researchers from the University of California, Berkeley, found that by up-regulating SIRT3 activity (which usually declines with age), they could reverse some of the markers of aging. Most importantly, increasing SIRT3 activity improves the ability of hematopoietic stem cells to regenerate. The researchers unambiguously said that *"aging-associated degeneration can be reversed by a sirtuin"*.

A commercially available drug that targets either SIRT1 or SIRT3 is a while away, however sirtuin-related therapy appears to be one of the most promising areas of current research into delaying or reversing the aging process.

No one has quite "nailed it" yet

Despite the abundance of theories, each with a varying degree of plausibility, no single theory has yet completely nailed down a single reason for exactly why animals age. This is most likely because aging will turn out to be underpinned by a range of different causes.

It is in the area of evolutionary theories in particular, where there are a range of confounding factors that makes it hard to make a convincing case for any single theory. For example, we have the basic theory that aging is helpful for a species as it clears out the weaker, elderly specimens, while preserving the younger generation, making the group as a whole, stronger. However there is an equally convincing case to be made that if we didn't age, we could continue to reproduce ad infinitum. Surely this would lead to greater numbers and therefore a stronger overall group would it not? Or would this just lead to a population explosion (like a rabbit plague, for example) which would deplete resources and lead to the implosion of the group or species? And could you not also say that by allowing the elderly to breed you are increasing the risk of genetic mutations being passed on, if you accept that an organism accumulates transmittable mutations?

Female menopause, on a particular level, appears to give us some indication of how evolution views aging and breeding. On an evolutionary level, menopause appears to exist with the single purpose of preventing an elderly person from reproducing and potentially not being able to care for her young. However this is then confounded by the fact that many species continue to breed for their entire life span.

And if evolution has set up aging as a mechanism to clear out *dead wood* (sorry to sound so clinical), why do so many females live so far past the time where they are fertile? Surely evolution would have set us up like spawning salmon, where we swim upstream to breed and then keel over dead. Salmon are a much better example of evolution only caring about breeding and not life span. But there are too many exceptions for this to be considered a genuine rule of thumb or guiding principle.

Then we have the problem of how different animals age at different rates. If there was a single, underlying factor driving the aging process, surely animals would all age at the same rate. If this was the case, a large dog that was roughly the same weight as a small person would have roughly the same life span. However we know this to not be the case, which is why we have the concept of *dog years*. The maximum life expectancy for a dog is around 15 or 16 years, whereas a human can often reach 80 years. Why do dogs wear out more quickly than humans?

If it was a question of weight, then surely similar animals would age at the same rate due to similar metabolism, heart rate etc. However this argument falls down in far too many examples to be of use. A rat usually lives to 3, while a chipmunk can reach 14. Humans are bigger than smaller animals so maybe we age more slowly for this reason. However smaller dogs live longer than bigger dogs and humans live almost twice as long as bears. There is not consistent theme here, so I think this is not an area of great potential for us to focus research efforts.

One concept that is a little more consistently applicable is the link between life span and sexual maturity. There does appear to be a link between these two factors. For example, animals that reach sexual maturity more quickly and produce larger numbers of offspring at a time, tend to have shorter life spans. So, is the relatively long life of a human linked to the time we take to reach sexual maturity and the fact that we only (usually) produce one offspring at a time? Maybe evolution tries to keep animals who breed slowly alive longer so they will have a better chance of creating enough progeny to repopulate. And why exactly do humans take so long to reach sexual maturity? Is it to allow females to grow wide enough hips to give birth to our relatively brain-heavy babies? Or is it because humans lack natural predators, giving us the luxury of taking our time to breed? Scientists have often noted that prey animals breed more quickly than predators, so perhaps they need to rush a little so they are not eaten before they have a chance to reproduce.

It is far too easy to get completely lost in theory here and miss the key point - *Irrespective of why we age, what can we do to increase our chances of reaching 100 and beyond?* That is the focus of the second part of this book.

Part 2 – How to live to 100 and beyond

So now that we are familiar with the various mechanisms that underlie the aging process, we need to apply what we know to increase our potential longevity. However, just tackling the cellular process that drive aging would be far too narrow. What would be the point of taking every anti-aging supplement under the sun if you go ahead and smoke cigarettes or live on junk food?

Therefore, if we are to take a holistic approach to increasing your chances of living to 100, we need to follow a range of general principles so we can tick of each of the factors that encourage a long life and each of the factors that has the chance to strike us down ahead of our time.

Now, let's look at each of these, one by one.

Prevent and reverse oxidative damage

If we are to accept that free radical damage (particularly from reactive oxygen species) is at least part of the cause of the aging process, the next question must be - *how do we stop or reverse this damage?* The answer, as you probably know, is primarily through antioxidants. Think of antioxidants as your fire fighters putting out the fire. However, shouldn't we also endeavor to stop lighting fires? Or, put another way, logically shouldn't we also try to ensure that we do all we can to minimize the creation of free radicals in the first place?

Unfortunately, due to the fact that a large component of free radical generation is unavoidable as a part of oxygen-based metabolism, we are limited in what we can do to minimal the production of them. In fact, after trawling through various research papers and journals, the only credible way I could find to reliably minimize the production of free radicals was to avoid marathon running and minimize UV exposure.

The "marathon running" one usually comes as a shock to people who have been conditioned to view long distance running as a super-healthy activity. Unfortunately this is not the case. Exercise always involves the generation of extra free radicals as a by-product of the ramped-up metabolic processes involved. Usually your body can deal with this extra production of free radicals and this effect is more than offset by the myriad of health benefits you get from cardiovascular exercise. However in the case of regular long distance running, there is such as massive spike in the production of free radicals that your body finds it difficult to keep up in its efforts to neutralize them. This is not new information. For many years now, long distance runners have been instructed to ramp up their consumption of antioxidants such as vitamin C, to help them offset this phenomenon.

Unfortunately for you running buffs out there, the science is turning against long distance running. Various studies have shown that high-intensity interval training (HIIT) tops long distance, steady-state running on just about any metric, from joint wear & tear to fat burning efficiency (i.e. - you can burn more calories in a much shorter period of time).

If running is your passion and it makes you happy (and doesn't ruin your joints), make sure you consume massive amounts of antioxidants through your diet and supplementation.

Anyway, more on this in the Exercise section.

So clearly, our best option for reducing and reversing oxidative damage is via diet and supplementation. But what is the difference between various antioxidants and how do we measure the ability of a substance to neutralize free radicals?

There are so many different antioxidants that I could bore you to death by literally filling an entire book trying to list them all. So instead, I want to focus on the most important and ubiquitous of the antioxidants. But first, let's get a better understanding of how we determine antioxidant capabilities.

How do you determine the antioxidant ability of a particular food?
The globally standardized method for assessing the ability of a substance to scavenge free radicals is a test measuring *oxygen radical absorbance capacity* (ORAC). So a food with a high ORAC score is considered to be high in antioxidant activity.

Whilst the ORAC number gives us a rough guide to antioxidant activity, there is no proven link between an ORAC score and a particular biological benefit. Many scientists believe that the ORAC score of a particular food is meaningless, whereas others believe it still has value as a general guiding principle.

However, if you acknowledge the importance of dietary antioxidants in preventing and reversing oxidative damage, as a general guide, the ORAC score of a particular food is as good as any for informing your understanding. Many people are vehemently opposed to even acknowledging the existence of the ORAC system because of the inherent flaws. They quite rightly point to the fact that there is often little correlation between chemical reactions in a test tube (in-vitro) and what happens in the human body. Also, the ORAC score takes into consideration only one aspect of antioxidant activity. However, my position is that, as long as you consider the ORAC score to be a guide to rough antioxidant activity and not accurate gospel, I have no problems with people trying to include more high ORAC foods into their diets.

Here are the ORAC values for some common* foods -

Dark Chocolate 20,823

Pecans 17,940

Walnuts 13,541

Hazelnuts 9,645

Cranberries, raw 9,584

Artichokes 9,416

Kidney beans, red 8,459

Pink beans 8,320

Black beans 8,040

Pistachio nuts 7,983

Currants 7,960

Pinto beans 7,779

Plums 7,581

Milk chocolate 7,528

Lentils 7,282

Dried apples 6,681

Blueberries 6,552

Prunes 6,552

Soybeans 5,764

Blackberries 5,347

Raw garlic 5,346

Cabernet Sauvignon (red wine variety) 5,034**

Raspberries 4,882

Almonds 4,454

Apples, red delicious 4,275

White raisins 4,188

Dates 3,895

Strawberries 3,577

Peanut butter 3,432

Red currants 3,387

Figs 3,383

Cherries 3,365

Gooseberries 3,277

Dried apricots 3,234

Peanuts 3,166

Red cabbage 3,145

Broccoli 3,083

Apples 3,082

Raisins 3,037

Pears 2,941

Guava 2,550

Red leaf lettuce 2,380

*Note - I have removed obscure foods from above and just focused on widely available, everyday foods.

** - I know what you are thinking. Don't even think about it!

In terms of pure ORAC punchiness, certain herbs and spices have numbers which dwarf everyday foods. However we tend to use much less quantity, so you need to take that into consideration. However this also shows the importance of eating "real" food. You will never find turmeric or cloves in a Big Mac.

Cloves 314,446

Cinnamon 267,536

Oregano 200,129

Turmeric 159,277

Vitamin C

As the most well-known and understood of the antioxidants, vitamin C provides a natural kick-off point for us to look at the different antioxidants. One of the things that primates (including man) have different to other mammals is that we cannot produce vitamin c (ascorbic acid) endogenously - we need to take it in through our diet. Vitamin C is a powerful scavenger of free radicals such as hydrogen peroxide, one of the most potentially damaging free radicals.

Fortunately a healthy diet rich in fruits and vegetables is likely to have good levels of vitamin c. A clinical vitamin c deficiency (scurvy, which, in times past would afflict sailors who did not have ready access to fresh food) is therefore relatively rare in the western world. However there is a massive gap between the minimum amount needed to avoid scurvy and the amount needed to prevent oxidative damage.

As well as treating oxidative stress, vitamin C is vital for a range of important reactions in the body and brain, such as the production on certain neurotransmitters and hormones.

In general I prefer to get vitamin c from food rather than supplements, however I am a fruit fanatic so this is not hard for me. If, for whatever reason, you can't get your vitamin C from food, then supplementation is the next best thing.

I would aim for a minimum of 500mg each day, in divided doses because vitamin C, being water soluble, cannot be stored in the body. Some of the foods highest in vitamin C include - peppers (capsicum), citrus fruit, kiwi fruit, guava, leafy green vegetables and berries.

In general, vitamin C is perfectly safe, with a couple of exceptions applying to supplements only. If vitamin C gives you gastrointestinal distress, stick to buffered types of vitamin C such as *calcium ascorbate*. Also, if you have been diagnosed with cancer and are currently undergoing treatment, only take vitamin C (or any other supplement at all) with your doctor's permission. There are certain scenarios where taking antioxidants during cancer treatment can have a paradoxically pro-oxidant effect.

Vitamin E

Vitamin E is actually a single term for a collection of various fat-soluble compounds that protect cells from free radical damage. Vitamin E is important in a different way to the water-soluble vitamin C, as it also targets the free radicals that are produced as a by-product of fat oxidation. As we heard earlier, oxidized LDL is one of the most damaging types of free radicals. The other piece of good news is that vitamin E and vitamin C act synergistically, both playing a role (a kind of "one-two punch" act) in neutralizing the same free radical molecule.

As with vitamin C, the benefits of vitamin E for conferring longevity benefits are not limited to free radical scavenging. Vitamin E has long been promoted as a "heart-healthy" supplement because it makes your arterial walls less sticky and inhibits platelet aggregation, both implicated in heart disease.

In general, as vital as vitamin E is, the evidence for its use as a supplement is not yet compelling enough. Or, put another way, a little bit of vitamin E in the diet is great, with more not necessarily better.

My favorite sources for vitamin E are nuts and avocado, both "super-foods" in their own right. Remember though – peanuts are not nuts (although they are indeed high in Vitamin E).

Astaxanthin

As if you didn't need another reason to take krill oil.

Krill oil contains a super-potent carotenoid antioxidant called *astaxanthin*, which appears to have significantly greater free radical scavenging activity than vitamin C and vitamin E. This appears to be linked to its ability to donate electrons (and thereby neutralizing free radicals) and continue to function, due to its surplus of electrons. As you will remember from earlier, typically an antioxidant will be broken down and recycled once it has done its job of donating an electron to a free radical. Most antioxidant molecules can also only deal with one free radical molecule at a time, whereas astaxanthin can neutralize a large number of free radicals simultaneously by surrounding them in an *electron cloud*. When I first read about how astaxanthin functions, I imagined that it must look like a kind of "antioxidant terminator" as it annihilates any free radical in its path.

Astaxanthin has recently been the subject of increasing interest and excitement from medical researchers due to the wide range of potential benefits it confers, such as reducing inflammation and preventing free radical damage in the eyes.

However its ability to protect the brain and cardiovascular system is where the bulk of recent research has been focused. It appears to have a particularly prominent ability to fight cognitive decline in the elderly by neutralizing phospholipid hydroperoxides, one of the hypothesized causes of Alzheimer's disease. In terms of cardiovascular effects, it appears to lower blood pressure, decrease triglycerides and increase HDL levels.

Another massive benefit over other carotenoids (such as beta carotene), is that in high doses, astaxanthin retains its antioxidant effects. Other carotenoids can become pro-oxidant in high doses. One of the reasons why it is not recommended to ever supplement with vitamin A or beta-carotene.

The best sources of astaxanthin are krill oil supplements and wild-caught salmon. Astaxanthin is what gives each of these their pinky-red color. This bears repeating - krill oil should be a compulsory addition to your anti-aging arsenal. It is as close as we get to a miracle pill.

Polyphenols and Flavonoids

I am not particularly enamored with reductionist thinking, as it tends to be overly simplistic. Like when you are told that depression is "caused by low serotonin" or that a particular food is healthy simply because it is high in vitamin C.

Likewise, any attempts to isolate the anti-aging benefits of various fruits and vegetables down to a single vitamin or mineral would be misguided.

The perfect example of this is when we look at the various polyphenols and flavonoids that certain fruit and vegetables contain. Simply isolating one of these particular substances and putting it into a pill rarely demonstrates the same health effects as just eating a piece of fruit.

Flavonoids (which are a type of polyphenol, or polyphenolic compound) have been the subject of considerable excitement in recent years. Have you noticed all those reports detailing the health benefits of green tea, blueberries and red wine? These are largely related to the various flavonoids that each of these foods (and drinks) contains.

One of the reasons why I feel the focus on single vitamins in food is misguided is that each day (assuming you eat a healthy diet) your consumption of various flavonoids far outweighs your consumption of, for example, vitamin C. Flavonoids are one of the reasons why you should be excited about fruits and vegetables and maximize your consumption of them.

One of the beauties of flavonoids is that they can target different aspects of oxidative stress concurrently. Depending on which particular flavonoid we are talking about, they can target not only oxidized LDL but also reactive oxygen species such as hydrogen peroxide as well.

Flavonoids are potent antioxidants that you should endeavor to make part of your daily diet. Don't worry about popping any particular pill. If you have a diet rich in multi-colored fruits and vegetables you should have most of your bases covered. The reason for the multi-colored requirement is that various flavonoids and polyphenols have different colors, so if you included a wide range of colors in your diet, you are almost certainly getting broad-spectrum antioxidant coverage.

However there are certain foods and drinks that have a particularly potent concentration of powerful flavonoids. You should try to include the following into your diet where possible -

Tea

A perfect example of the reason why it is difficult to be reductionist about the health effects of certain foods is good old fashioned tea (*camellia Sinensis*). Not only does tea contain potent antioxidants known as *catechins*, it also contains L-theanine, an amino acid that has relaxation-inducing and mood-brightening effects.

The main catechin found in tea is called *epigallocatechin gallate* (EGCG) and is found mostly in green tea and white tea (black tea loses a lot of the catechin activity due to the extra processing step needed). EGCG has been found in various animal and laboratory studies to inhibit the development of certain cancers. However it should be pointed out that this was under mega-dosing conditions - far in excess of the levels you would get from drinking tea. Some companies are now working on developing concentrated forms of EGCG as a potential cancer preventative or treatment.

However, in the meantime, the ability of EGCG to work as an antioxidant is not disputed.

Tea would be considered a "super-food" simply based on its catechin content, however the good news doesn't stop there. Green tea is also a potent *thermogenic* (it increases metabolic rate, leading to potential fat loss). If we accept that overweight and obesity are a major driver of premature mortality, this must also be considered as a factor in evaluating tea's longevity-promoting effects.

Another bonus is the L-theanine content I just mentioned. L-theanine has been shown to increase levels of dopamine and to a lesser extent, serotonin, in the brain. Unsurprisingly, L-theanine is now a popular supplement for those needing a mood-boost or sleep improvement.

Berries

One of the main reasons why you would have seen blueberries plastered around everywhere as a "super-food" is because they contain a potent flavonoid known as *anthocyanin*. This flavonoid, which gives berries their dark red and purple color, has been shown to potently inhibit the oxidation of fats. A study published in the *Journal of Biomedicine and Biotechnology* found that anthocyanin had a beneficial effect on the cardiovascular system by preventing lipid oxidation. Another study conducted by the U.S. Department of Agriculture's Human Nutrition Research Center on Aging at Tufts University, found that anthocyanin ameliorated age-related losses of cognitive function in rodents.

Another reason to include liberal amounts of berries in your diet is that they are relatively low in fructose. Despite what you may have read, fruit should not be consumed in unlimited amounts. At a certain point, the antioxidant benefits will be outweighed by the damaging effects of fructose. This can be mitigated to a certain extent by focusing on low-fructose fruits such as berries.

Resveratrol

One exception to my usual rule of focusing on real foods as your main source of antioxidants is resveratrol. This is because the most common source of resveratrol that people focus on is red wine. Anything up to a third of a glass of red wine per day is net-positive for your health, however if you go beyond this, the negative effects of alcohol will outweigh the benefits of the extra resveratrol.

Over the past few years, resveratrol has become the darling of the life-extension community due to some interesting research results. Studies have shown the ability to lengthen telomeres, reduce blood sugar, reduce inflammation and even extend the life of certain basic organisms such as fruit flies and worms. Similarly, a study on fish showed a significant life-span enhancing effect (more than 50%) with resveratrol.

Various cancer-related studies have also shown that, in certain situations, resveratrol has the ability to either prevent cancer or reduce the size of existing cancers. This is all preliminary research however, so please do not view resveratrol as a proven cancer-fighter just yet until more research is available.

In the brain, resveratrol has also been shown to reduce the formation of *beta-amyloid plaque*, which is thought to be the main cause of Alzheimer's disease. Again, this is all preliminary stuff, although interesting and promising nonetheless.

In terms of the alcohol issue, the way I look at it is - if you are determined to drink alcohol, at least stick to red wine to get the modest cardio-protective and resveratrol-related benefits. However please do not fool yourself by thinking you are extending your life-span by chugging cheap pinot noir every night.

A much better option is to take a resveratrol supplement. These usually contain resveratrol from the world's richest known source - *Japanese knotweed*.

Glutathione – The "master antioxidant"

Inside your body there is a simple molecule which you have possibly never heard of, yet is integral to both your physical health and the speed at which you age. This molecule is *glutathione*. It is so important that it is sometimes referred to as the *master antioxidant* or the *mother of all antioxidants*. This is not just hyperbole either. I will get to why in a moment.

Due to the fact that glutathione contains organically bonded sulfur (via the amino acids that make up glutathione), glutathione is the most powerful single way to reduce oxidative stress and detoxify. Sulfur is a sticky molecule that binds to reactive oxygen species and certain toxins, rendering them inactive.

Often in natural health books or websites, you will read the term "detoxify" in vague, nebulous ways. You will hear that sweating helps you detoxify (it doesn't - you don't eliminate toxins via the skin) or that you need to go on a "detox diet". Rarely will you even be told what these nefarious "toxins" are. However, as I pointed out in my guides on milk thistle and liver detoxification supplements, there are occasions where the term "detoxify" is apt. Typically these occasions refer to increasing the ability of your liver to detoxify various substances (such as acetaminophen, which I will get to in a moment) and by increasing levels of glutathione.

The most powerful example of why glutathione is so important is the case of acetaminophen (paracetamol in certain countries) overdose. If you or one of your pets takes a massive dose of acetaminophen, left untreated it will often lead to liver failure and then death. The reason for this is that your liver uses glutathione to neutralize acetaminophen, which is a harmful toxin for your body. After receiving a massive dose of acetaminophen, you literally run out of glutathione, leading to the accumulation of acetaminophen in your liver. At a certain point your liver then shuts down.

This is how important glutathione is.

However where this gets truly interesting is when we look at one of the treatments for acetaminophen overdose. This substance also happens to be my number one supplement for optimizing glutathione levels - *N-acetylcysteine*. Yes, the same substance given intravenously to overdose patients is also available as an over the counter (OTC) supplement.

Importantly, glutathione is not just vital as an antioxidant in its own right, it also functions to boost the effectiveness of other antioxidants such as vitamin C, vitamin E and lipoic acid.

As glutathione levels gradually decrease as you age, it has been suggested as one of the central players in the aging process and certain diseases associated with age.

Unfortunately you can't just take glutathione as a pill, so the only way to increase levels is to take in the precursors of glutathione via your diet or supplementation. The easiest way to boost levels via your diet is to consume foods rich in precursor amino acids such as cysteine (which contains sulfur). The best foods for this are cruciferous vegetables such as broccoli, along with sulfur-rich foods such as garlic or onions.

However the most powerful single way to increase levels of glutathione is by supplementation. Here are my picks for supplements that boost glutathione levels -

N-acetylcysteine (NAC)

As I mentioned earlier, NAC has a long history of use in medicine - particularly for the treatment of acute paracetamol (acetaminophen) overdose and for breaking up the thick mucus associated with conditions such as cystic fibrosis.

In recent years, due to the wide range of beneficial effects that NAC has on the body, it has become increasingly popular as a supplement. All too often, the latest 'buzz' supplement turns out to be mostly hot air. However, NAC is one substance where I can vouch for its powerful and positive effects on the liver and brain. Interestingly, NAC is also one supplement where both the 'natural health' people and the medical community are in agreement. I was reminded of this the other day when a friend visited a specialist for fibromyalgia. As well as several different pain and sleep medications, the specialist had also recommended a daily dose of NAC. It is not often you leave a specialist's office with a recommendation to take supplements!

What is NAC?

NAC is closely related to the amino acid cysteine, with a few minor chemical differences. This does not really tell us much about it at all, so it is best to discuss what it does rather than what it is. And the best way to look at that is to refer back to why NAC is used for paracetamol overdose.

As I previously mentioned, an overdose of paracetamol depletes the liver of glutathione which is needed to clear the toxic levels of the drug from your body. This kind of overdose is the most common cause of acute liver failure in the US today. NAC is one of the most potent agents available for increasing glutathione.

Remember, NAC has the support of both the alternative medicine and the scientific community. According to Stanford University's Dr. Kondala R. Atkuri, "NAC has been used successfully to treat glutathione deficiency in a wide range of infections, genetic defects and metabolic disorders, including HIV infection and Chronic Obstructive Pulmonary Disease. Over *two-thirds of 46 placebo-controlled clinical trials with orally administered NAC have indicated beneficial effects of NAC measured either as trial endpoints or as general measures of improvement in quality of life and well-being of the patients."*

For example, a trial with results published in the November 2006 journal *Apoptosis*, looked at whether NAC could stop or reverse liver cell death in subjects with life-threatening liver failure. Based on results with animal test subjects, researchers reached the conclusion that NAC showed a clear liver-protective benefit in this situation. Another study which was published in the January 2008 edition of the journal *Liver Transplantation*, found that children who received NAC for acute liver failure had a better survival rates and positive health outcomes than those not receiving NAC.

Apart from its use in emergency wards to prevent liver failure, NAC is also used for a wide range of other illnesses and diseases –

* NAC has been shown to protect against some strains of influenza

* NAC is sometimes used to treat chronic obstructive pulmonary disease (COPD)

* NAC has been shown reduce oxidative stress caused by exercise (note - this doesn't mean that exercise is bad for you - it means that intense or long duration exercise can increase some types of harmful oxidative stress)

* NAC improves insulin sensitivity in patients with type 2 diabetes or other forms of insulin resistance and metabolic derangement.

* NAC has been shown to improve both schizophrenia and bipolar disorder. However at this stage, the mechanism of action remains unclear. It is believed that one of the main reasons is that NAC modulates NMDA receptors and the overall level of glutamate in the brain. However this is not yet proven and there could be another mechanism of action at work.

* NAC has been used to treat marijuana and cocaine addiction with success

* NAC is often used on HIV patients due to its immune-stimulating effects

* NAC can be used to chelate (detoxify) the body of heavy metals such as mercury and also prevent damage to internal organs such as the kidneys, by mercury and other heavy metals.

* NAC has also been trialed as a treatment for *Sjogren's syndrome*. NAC was shown to reduce eye pain in a recent study.

* NAC has also been shown to act as a potent anti-inflammatory due to the reduction of oxidative stress (due to its antioxidant action) and also its ability to reduce levels of pro-

inflammatory substances in the body such as *IL-6 (interleukin 6)*. Remember, widespread inflammation puts additional stress on the liver.

* Due to both its antioxidant and anti-inflammatory actions, along with other mechanisms of action such as preventing DNA damage, NAC has been shown to inhibit the development of various cancers.

* NAC has been shown to increase release of the neurotransmitter dopamine and protect against the damage of dopamine receptors in the brain from chronic amphetamine use.

* NAC has been shown to dramatically decrease levels of *lipoprotein (a)*. A recent trial showed that oral NAC decreased levels of lipoprotein (a) by 70%. High levels of Lipoprotein (a) have been associated with increased risk of heart disease, so by bringing down levels of lipoprotein (a) NAC has shown some promise in this area.

Alpha lipoic acid – The fat & water-soluble powerhouse

Alpha lipoic acid (ALA) is a compound produced in the body which acts as a co-factor for the production of vital energy from the metabolism of branched-chain amino acids. This energy production occurs at the cellular level – in our mitochondria, which we were familiar with from earlier in the book. In this respect, ALA works at the same level as another very important co-factor - co-enzyme Q10 (*Co-Q10* or *ubiquinone*). Think back to science class and how chemical reactions require different agents. In your body, substances such as ALA and Co-Q10 are necessary for certain energy-producing reactions.

ALA acts as an antioxidant by scavenging various reactive oxygen species (ROS) and is one of the only antioxidants that is both water and fat soluble. Antioxidants are typically either one or the other and therefore have a mode of action in specific parts of the body. For example, Vitamin C is water soluble but not fat soluble, whereas Vitamin E and Vitamin A are fat soluble, not water soluble. Often the best way to tell is by the tablet they come in. Vitamin E and A usually come in transparent gel caps (like fish oil tables), whereas Vitamin C is usually a powder or tablet made from powder. ALA is not just water and fat soluble - it also recycles other antioxidants and similar substances such as Vitamin E, Co-Q10 and glutathione.

ALA's ability to scavenge free radicals has been backed up by extensive testing which has shown that ALA decreases urinary *isoprostanes*, *oxidized LDL* and *plasma protein carbonyls*, which are biomarkers of oxidative stress in the body. I should also point out that oxidized LDL is one of the strongest known factors in the potential development of heart disease via inflammation of the arteries.

Also, it is important to note that, like N-acetylcysteine, ALA is not just a substance limited to the world of alternative health. In countries such as Germany, ALA is a recognized gold-standard treatment for various neuropathies (nerve pain disorders) such as diabetic neuropathy, due primarily to its ability to increase aortic blood flow. This bears emphasizing - ALA is a substance with documented, identifiable and beneficial effects on the human body.

Despite the range of beneficial effects that ALA has on the body, it is the ability of ALA to recycle and increase levels of glutathione that for me is of most interest in the context of anti-aging.

Despite the body of evidence, ALA as a means to increase levels of glutathione is taking longer to catch on than more well-known substances such as NAC or milk thistle. And this is not due to a lack of studies - in fact the first major human trial was conducted way back in the 1970s by the National Institutes of Health (NIH). The results of even this very first trial were amazing - out of 79 people with severe liver damage, 75 recovered full liver function after a period using ALA. As recently as 1999, there was a follow up trial by the same researchers using a combination of ALA, silymarin (milk thistle) and selenium in patients with liver disease. All patients recovered liver function and did not require subsequent transplants - a remarkable result when you consider how little-known this substance is. The mechanism by which this was achieved was through the glutathione boosting effect.

Selenium

Selenium is a trace element that plays an important function assisting glutathione in neutralizing free radicals such as hydrogen peroxide. More specifically, selenium is a co-factor in the production of glutathione peroxidase, which targets and neutralizes reactive oxygen species such as hydrogen peroxide.

Selenium is another classic example of "little is good, too much is very bad", as it is toxic in high doses. Selenium is not something I recommend you supplement with. If you eat a healthy diet with a wide range of different foods, you are unlikely to be deficient.

There have been a range of studies that implicate selenium deficiency in a wide range of conditions such as cancer and diabetes, however actual trials have failed to show any benefit for selenium supplementation.

However, others believe that selenium deficiency is more common than is currently reported. Renowned author of _"The Four-Hour Body"_, Tim Ferriss, is one example of someone who discovered that they had a selenium deficiency. In Ferriss's case, it manifested in the form of low testosterone, so, when he fixed his selenium deficiency, his testosterone status normalized.

If you suspect a selenium deficiency, you can easily get it tested. Just request this test with your doctor. However a much easier option is to religiously eat two Brazil nuts every day. That should give you just the right amount of selenium for optimal functioning.

Do I need to take supplements?

In terms of your own requirements for supplementation, you should be guided by -

- Your probable level of oxidative stress and toxin insult. If you consume a lot of alcohol and junk food, smoke, or are in environments with high levels of toxins (such as China and the airborne mercury issue), you will need more.

- Your consumption of sulfur rich foods such as cruciferous vegetables, onions and garlic. If you eat a diet high in sulfur rich foods, you may need less supplementation support.

- Your genetics. Some people have impaired function of the GSTM1 gene, which is required for normal glutathione activity. These people need to supplement to provide additional support to their glutathione synthesis pathway.

Healthy weight

How many obese 80 year olds do you see? If you think back to all the centenarians you have seen on television being celebrated for reaching this important milestone, what was their typical body type? All pretty thin weren't they?

Not only does being overweight dramatically increase your chance of dying by cardiovascular disease and certain types of cancers, it triggers a range of biological changes that age you more quickly than those at a healthy weight. Not only does being overweight expose you directly to increased mortality, it causes primary illnesses that can then lead to early death or accelerated aging. Type 2 diabetes is a classic example of this. At a cellular level, getting type 2 diabetes is like stepping into an aging acceleration machine.

Recently, scientists have identified clear links between body fat percentage and cellular aging. For example a recent study which looked at more than a thousand women of various ages found that as the body weight increased, telomere length shortened. This is believed to be driven by levels of the hunger/satiety hormone *leptin* which is stored in fat cells. The higher the level of leptin, the shorter the telomere. As an aside, the same study also found that smokers have shorter telomeres than non-smokers. But that's not particularly surprising right? Nothing surprising there. What is more surprising is that being overweight was associated with shorter telomeres than smoking was! Now that I found surprising.

A study published in 2009 in the journal Nature, found that *"Obesity accelerates the aging of adipose tissue, a process only now beginning to come to light at the molecular level. Experiments in mice suggest that obesity increases the formation of reactive oxygen species in fat cells, shortens telomeres—and ultimately results in activation of the p53 tumor suppressor, inflammation and the promotion of insulin resistance."*

No one wants to reach 100 and have no quality of life, and one of the biggest factors in quality of life is mobility. Lacking mobility dramatically reduces the activities you can enjoy as you get older. Not to mention the fact that extended periods sitting down is associated with lower life expectancy. Also key is the disturbing tendency of people to suddenly go downhill and die soon after breaking a hip in old age.

Being overweight is extremely taxing on your skeletal system and increases your chances of suffering from various forms of osteoarthritis. This is compounded by the fact that being overweight itself, reduces your ability to engage in the kinds of healthy exercise that helps protect against arthritis later in life.

However it is important to note that more isn't always better. If there is on consistent point I like to make is that you should always look for balance. If we look at the other end of the spectrum from overweight people, we will find ex-athletes. It is one of the great tragedies of competitive sport that when athletes retire, they are often struck down from various injuries that have come from a life of over-use. Particularly bad is the arthritis that often sets in where there has been a previous injury sustained - such as knee ligaments.

So where possible, if you plan on leading a long life of optimal mobility, your focus needs to be on low-impact exercises. One of the most hotly debated topics in physical fitness at the moment is the recent understanding that long-distance running is actually net-negative due to both the spectacularly high level of oxidative stress and the negative effects on the joints of many years of long-distance running. Previously, marathon running was held up as a paragon of healthy living, until healthy professionals started pointing out that they were seeing a lot of long-distance runners with knees and ankles completely shot.

Fortunately, we now know that you can achieve the positive health benefits of exercise with much less strain on your joints by either engaging in low impact exercise or focusing on high intensity interval training (HIIT - as mentioned in the section on exercise). Researchers have found that the same weight loss benefits can be achieved with short periods of intense exercise, compared to long periods pounding the pavement at a medium intensity (this type of exercise is called steady-state exercise as the intensity stays roughly consistent during each session). The way they measure this is by putting them on a bike and measuring their *VO2 max* (also known as *maximal aerobic capacity*), which is a fairly reliable measure of energy expenditure.

Therefore, to ensure that you get the benefits of exercise without putting undue wear and tear on your musculoskeletal system, the following types of exercise could be a good starting point. Note that I have included yoga below. Unless doing intense forms of *Ashtanga* yoga or some of the more advanced *Iyengar* series of poses, yoga is generally not a particularly effective form of cardiovascular work. However, what it does have going for it, is the unrivalled ability to improve mobility. You can see this when you see elderly yoga adepts, who move like someone significantly younger than they are. However in the interests of balance I should also mention a counterpoint to the argument that yoga prevents injury. Some experts in physiology believe that yoga can also be harmful as it increases range of motion to such as degree that there is an increased risk of hyper-extension related injuries. Even if this was correct, I think it applies to a small subset of the population who are doing very heavy lifting in the weights room.

Here are some potential options for suitable forms of exercise -

- Swimming

- Yoga

- Pilates

- Cycling

- Ping-Pong (also excellent for building hand-eye co-ordination)

- Weight training (it's no use being in shape if you have no muscles supporting your skeletal system)

- Walking

- Rowing

- Rollerblading (chance of injury however)

- Water aerobics

Before I go, I need to point out one more thing. Being underweight is also not healthy. Sorry to bang on about it however the key is balance. When you are dramatically underweight, your body assumes that you are in a famine and undergoes a variety of processes. The most obvious of which is that in dangerously thin women, their menstruation stops. And this is not just limited to the painfully thin. New research suggests that someone with excellent muscle definition due to low body-fat percentage is also not the ideal. Your body needs some body fat as an energy buffer and for various biological processes. A little bit of body fat is good, too much is very, very bad.

Reduce inflammation

In terms of supplements that reduce levels inflammation in the body, there are two which I consider virtually compulsory - omega 3 fatty acids and curcumin. While both are potent anti-inflammatories, they operate via different pathways, with a range of consequent benefits throughout the body.

Omega 3 Fatty Acids

Like several other important nutrients and supplements, a testament to the body-wide benefits of omega 3 is the fact that I could have included it in a number of sections, from the brain to the cardiovascular system. However I believe that it is one particular mechanism that drives the majority of all the omega 3-related benefits - its ability to switch the body from a *pro*-inflammatory to an *anti*-inflammatory state. To learn why it does this, we will need to also look at omega 6 fatty acids and the sometimes yin-yang relationship between these two vital fats.

Omega 3, in the form of fish oil or krill oil tablets, along with the consumption of healthy seafood, is one of the most important things you can do for your brain and body in terms of increasing longevity.

If we first look to the brain, one of the key factors that enables the quick and efficient transfer of information around your brain is the health of your myelin, which is a fatty sheath that covers your nerves. And yes, you guessed it, your myelin is essentially made of omega 3. You may have heard what happens when your myelin become damaged and dysfunctional - multiple sclerosis (MS), which is a debilitating, progressive neurological disorder. We do not yet know the cause of multiple sclerosis, however inflammation (and potentially vitamin D deficiency) is strongly implicated.

However it is omega 3's role as a potent anti-inflammatory that underlies most of the beneficial effects we see with this amazing fatty acid. In your brain and body, we can say (for illustration purposes) that inflammation is controlled by omega 6 (which increases inflammation) and Omega 3 (which decreases it). Remember, inflammation is not dangerous in itself - without inflammation your body would not be able to heal certain injuries and fight illness. The problems only emerge when the balance between omega 3 and omega 6 gets of out of whack. The theory as to why inflammation today runs rampant in humans is that in the past, our diets were more skewed to omega 3 rich foods. However today, with our grain-based diet, we consume far too much omega 6 and not enough omega 3. Not only do we consume a large amount of grain, our animals are now also mainly fed grains and oilseeds (corn, wheat, barley, soybean meal) instead of grass, so our meat is also now high in Omega 6.

The single best thing you can do to rectify this is to take a large dose of fish oil or krill oil. Certain research suggests that krill may be better absorbed and it also contains astaxanthin, so if your budget can stretch, I highly recommend krill supplements.

There is a fascinating area of research recently which hypothesizes that depression may be associated with elevated levels of inflammation in the brain. As this is early days, scientists don't yet know whether inflammation causes depression or whether depression causes inflammation, however it is certainly a promising line of inquiry. Due to the fact that many sufferers of depression have indicated that omega 3 appears to help them, this would make perfect sense.

My preference is to get your omega 3 from a wide-range of sources. Omega 3 contains two important substances - DHA (*docosahexaenoic acid*) and EPA (*eicosapentaenoic acid*). Each source of omega 3 has different ratios of these two substances and different levels of absorption by your body. The most common sources of omega 3 include - fish oil, krill oil, cod liver oil* (which also contains vitamin D and vitamin A), seafood** (particularly fatty fish), grass-fed beef and eggs.

Due to the fact that cod liver oil also contains Vitamin A, you should be careful to keep your consumption of this at reasonable levels. In some instances, high levels of Vitamin A can be toxic for humans. More is not always better.

** *Be careful to keep your consumption of certain fish that are high in mercury to sensible levels. In general, fish at the top of the food chain such as sharks, tuna or swordfish, are the main offenders you need to be careful of.*

Curcumin

One of the most exciting developments to come out of scientific research in recent years has been the growing understanding of the benefits of curcumin for the human body. Curcumin, which is extracted from turmeric (yes, the same turmeric used in Indian curries), has a long history in certain cultures for treating a range of complaints. The good news is that these traditional claims are now being backed up by rigorous, placebo-controlled clinical trials.

The range of effects that curcumin has on the body is surprisingly extensive, however most attention has been given to curcumin's abilities as an anti-inflammatory, anti-depressant and anti-cancer agent.

Firstly, what exactly is curcumin, and the turmeric plant from which it is extracted?

Turmeric, or curcuma longa, is a member of the ginger family. It is a perennial plant which grows to about 5-6 feet tall in the tropical regions of southern Asia. Turmeric has been used for over 4000 years both as a medicinal herb as well as a spice for cooking. It is fragrant, with a bitter and sharp character to taste.

It is made up of three main compounds; *desmethoxycurcumin, bis-desmethoxycurcumin* and *curcumin*, with curcumin being the most active *curcuminoid* of the turmeric plant and hence where the majority of attention is focused. In traditional medicine and naturopathic modalities, such as India's Ayurvedic system, turmeric has been used to treat a wide range of problems including arthritis, jaundice, heartburn (dyspepsia), stomach pain, diarrhea, intestinal gas, stomach bloating, appetite loss, liver issues, gallbladder disorders, laryngitis, bronchitis, diabetes, headaches, bronchitis, lung infections, fibromyalgia, colds, leprosy and cancer. Now, that is a pretty long list and naturally many of these traditional applications have not yet been verified by enough scientific evidence to be recommended by the medical community. There are quite a few studies already underway, looking to determine if curcumin demonstrates any ability to manage or treat arthritis, stomach ulcers, Alzheimer's disease and high cholesterol.

However, that doesn't mean that curcumin hasn't already been extensively studied. In PubMed (the database of various clinical trials), curcumin is cited almost 4000 times, with strong evidence to suggest effectiveness – as an antioxidant, anti-inflammatory, anti-atherosclerotic, preventing liver and kidney toxicity, as a potential treatment for psoriasis, diabetes, multiple sclerosis, Alzheimer's, HIV disease, septic shock, cardiovascular disease, lung fibrosis, arthritis, and inflammatory bowel disease!

That long list alone would be sufficient to justify further studies, however curcumin also shows in vitro (i.e. – in a test tube essentially, not in a human or animal subject) anti-cancer benefits, appearing to treat a number of cancers including breast, colon, kidney, liver, basal cell carcinoma, prostate, melanoma and also leukemia.

The single greatest negative health consequence of the modern-day inflammation epidemic is the incidence of heart disease. Many people do not realize that inflammation of the cardiovascular system is behind the majority of incidences of heart disease. For a long time, cholesterol has been the 'bad guy' – and unfairly so. Blaming cholesterol for heart disease is like blaming a fireman for a fire. The cholesterol is just there to put out the fire (inflammation).

However irrespective of what is causing inflamed arteries, curcumin is proving to be a potent treatment for arterial inflammation alongside other substances such as Omega 3 fatty acids. Various studies have shown that curcumin is able to suppress or reverse the effects of certain pro-inflammatory substances in the body such as *cytokines*.

Curcumin's benefit for the liver appears to be only slightly related to its potent anti-inflammatory properties. In terms of the liver, it is the fact that curcumin is a potent antioxidant and booster of glutathione levels which is behind the liver-healing effects of this amazing substance.

Clinical studies have shown that curcumin possesses the rare ability to massively boost your body's ability to produce glutathione and keep your liver in perfect condition (along with N-acetylcysteine, alpha lipoic acid and milk thistle). For example, researchers at the Medical University Graz in Austria revealed that curcumin as a compound delays the onset of liver damage caused by cirrhosis.

Curcumin has also been shown to boost the production of bile, assisting the liver in its efforts to digest dietary fat. The evidence has been sufficiently strong for the German Commission E (the scientific advisory board for Germany's equivalent of the Food & Drug Administration) to approves turmeric as a treatment for gastrointestinal problems.

Curcumin has stood up to a massive amount of testing to confirm its safety. Amazingly, it has been associated with no obvious toxic effects on the body. On the contrary, several studies have shown that administration of curcumin reduces the toxicity of other poisons such as arsenic.

If I was forced to imagine a potential downside, it could be in cases where some degree of inflammation is required and curcumin suppresses this. However, this scenario would be exceedingly rare. The human inflammation system is an 'over-reacting' system. This means that it usually creates inflammation far in excess of what is required, as, in evolutionary terms, this would be the better outcome for the body. As curcumin only reduces inflammation and doesn't eliminate it altogether, I would still think that there would be very few occasions where curcumin could be dangerous due to its anti-inflammatory properties.

As curcumin reduces clotting, it would be advisable to avoid curcumin leading up to any surgery, as the body's clotting ability is vital after any major procedure. Curcumin should not be taken along with blood thinners such as Warfarin and certain drugs used to treat diabetes, high cholesterol, stomach ulcers or high blood pressure.

Often other substances are added to curcumin supplements for certain reasons. Bromelain is sometimes added to increase the anti-inflammatory effect, however the majority of additives are included to increase bioavailability (the ability of your body to use the curcumin you take). Certain substances such as *piperine* increase the bioavailability of curcumin dramatically and thereby increasing the effectiveness of the dose you take. Curcumin has low bioavailability so if you are consuming, say, an Indian curry, your body is generally unable to take up much of the curcumin. In general, I like adding piperine supplements to my regime because many supplements (such as milk thistle) also suffer from low bioavailability. Alternatively, buy brands that combine the active agent with another substance (such as piperine) that increases bioavailability.

Curcumin for me is one of the most exciting supplements to come to prominence in recent times. Many herbs and supplements are either ineffective or too weak in comparison to any pharmaceutical options to be viable as treatments. Curcumin is no such supplement. Its effects are surprisingly potent – especially in the area of inflammation reduction. I believe inflammation is one of the largely undiagnosed epidemics of recent times, causing anything from cancer to heart disease.

There are not too many supplements out there that have positive effects on the brain, heart, liver, kidneys, stomach, joints and blood sugar. Curcumin is one such supplement.

Vitamin D

Vitamin D is another one that could be slotted into just about anywhere in this book. It is gradually become the nutritional version of the hottest Hollywood actor – everyone is talking about it. For years vitamin D was just that "thing" that people knew you "got from sunshine". However the latest research is indicating that Vitamin D is implicated a surprising array of health conditions that affect longevity.

However not only does vitamin D directly target inflammation, it also appears to directly target aging via inhibiting telomere shortening. It is believed to achieve this via its ability to inhibit pro-inflammatory processes. Vitamin D also inhibits certain kinds of dangerous cell proliferation mechanisms. For anyone out there with psoriasis, you would already be aware of this, as a vitamin D analogue called *calcipotriol* is a key ingredient in some anti-psoriasis creams, because it inhibits the cell proliferation associated with this particular skin condition.

A 2012 study which was published in the Journal of Immunology was able to clearly identify the cellular processes involved in vitamin D's inflammation-fighting abilities. The lead author concluded *"Patients with chronic inflammatory diseases, such as asthma, arthritis and prostate cancer, who are vitamin D deficient, may benefit from vitamin D supplementation to get their serum vitamin D levels above 30 nanograms/milliliter"*.

The latest recommendations are to get at least 20 minutes per day of direct sunlight on exposed sections of your body and to consider supplementing with vitamin D also. Remember that if you supplement with vitamin D, please ensure you also supplement with vitamin K to ensure that there are no cardiovascular complications from the extra vitamin D.

More controversial is the growing number of people who are experimenting with mega-doses of vitamin D. This goes against traditional advice regarding vitamin D toxicity, however some of these people are reporting startling improvements in a range of health complaints. It is too early to tell yet whether mega-dosing is a sensible practice, however what I can say with confidence is that the general recommendations for serum vitamin D levels and daily limits are too low. People such as the author of that particular book are consuming doses of vitamin D that doctors would consider toxic, yet are seeing a resolution of a range of illnesses. At the very least, this topic requires more research and a probable upwards revision of recommended daily levels.

When you visit the doctor to get a checkup and order certain tests, make sure you request a vitamin D test also. Some research suggests the majority of people in the western world are deficient due to avoidance of sunshine and changes in dietary habits from vitamin D-rich foods to grain-based junk food.

Prevent aging from sugar and AGEs

As we have already heard, AGEs are believed to play a central role in accelerated and premature cellular aging. So we therefore need to ensure we minimize consumption of AGEs or foods that trigger the production of AGEs. The single most powerful way to do this (and also address other factors in aging such as inflammation) is to minimize your consumption of sugar, and in particular, fructose. High levels of fructose consumption (and in particular, high-fructose corn syrup) promote both inflammation and the production of AGEs.

I like using extremes to illuminate potential issues with health and the best way to get an idea on why sugar ages you, we just have to look at what happens over time with diabetes. The elevated blood glucose levels associated with diabetes gradually ages and destroys parts of your body. The list of negative consequences of elevated blood sugar is long and extensive, however just a few of the problems include – diabetic neuropathy (where elevated blood glucose damages nerves), diabetic nephropathy (damage to kidneys from elevated blood sugar), diabetic retinopathy (damage to the retina from diabetes). From the same study published in *Nutrients* that I mentioned earlier in the book *"Accumulation of AGEs has been found in healthy aging persons, and this accumulation is higher during high glucose concentrations. Microvascular and macrovascular damage, seen in diabetes, is attributed to the accumulation of AGEs in tissues"*.

It's not the fat, but the 2.5 pounds of sugar that the average America consumes each week that is driving the obesity epidemic. This is because sugar (and other quick digesting carbohydrate bad-guys like bread and pasta) impair insulin and leptin sensitivity, directing your cells to store more energy as fat.

Put simply, if you want to get on top of inflammation, AGEs and the resultant acceleration of cellular aging, you have to minimize consumption of exogenous dietary AGEs and all forms of sugar.

One of the emerging theories on atherosclerosis and heart disease proposes that the formation of dangerous plaque in your arteries is largely causes by scarring caused as an unintended consequence of your immune system trying to neutralize AGEs.

Sugar is addictive and so dramatically cutting your consumption of sugar in a short space of time can result in all kinds of withdrawal effects, not unlike someone withdrawing from a street drug. Therefore, to maximize your chances of success, I suggest you gradually shift your diet away from sweeter flavors and back towards neutral or savory flavors.

The best example of this is sweetened beverages like coffee. Many people swear by the technique of gradually reducing the sugar you add to your hot drinks slowly enough so your taste buds don't notice. Like most people, when I was a child I could only tolerate tea or coffee with plenty of added sugar – a habit which usually carries over into adulthood for most. Nowadays, if I accidentally taste sweetened hot drinks, I find them intolerably sweet.

Your sense of taste tends to find a level of homeostasis based around your diet. If you consume a lot of sweets, you can tolerate sweeter food. If you eat a mainly savory diet, you tend to gravitate away from sweet food. The best way to see this in action is if you ever try a *ketogenic* diet for a few days. Ketogenic diets involve the consumption of almost no sweet foods or carbohydrates. In the absence of glucose, your body makes a kind of glucose proxy called *ketone bodies*, which your brain is able to use as a fuel source. The main benefit of this kind of diet is dramatic weight loss (again reinforcing why the best way to lose weight is to reduce carbohydrates and not fat). The interesting part happens when you reintroduce carbohydrates after the diet has ended. You will notice that a strange thing has happened to your taste buds – they have regained their sensitivity to sugar. Herein lies an extremely important point – if you find low-sugar diets difficult because you think you crave sweet flavors, you will soon adapt as your own taste buds adapt. Gradually, you will need less and less sugar to get that little mood-boost from foods on the sweet spectrum.

So what makes fructose so bad anyway? It all comes down to how your body processes fructose compared to glucose. Your body (and in particular, your brain) has a better ability to directly utilize glucose, whereas fructose must undergo a large proportion of its metabolism in the liver, where it is converted into free fatty acids, very low-density lipoprotein (VLDL – the type of cholesterol transporter that you *should* be worried about) and triglycerides. Not only are these substances known contributing factors for heart disease, they also tend to end up stored as fat.

Fructose has also been shown to interfere with leptin-mediated hunger signaling, making you feel less full and hungrier, which leads to greater weight accumulation.

It is one of the great modern-day tragedies that Americans have been subjected to the dietary horror that is *high-fructose corn syrup*. The American love affair with soda (which is largely sweetened with high-fructose corn syrup) is one of the major health emergencies facing its population.

Most Americans don't realize that in most other places around the world, high-fructose corn syrup is not widely used. Most countries sweeten commercially made products (such as sodas) using sucrose from cane sugar or sugar beets. For this, Americans have the good old USDA and Federal Government to thank. The various subsidies given to American farmers to grow corn, has led to frantic efforts to find uses for all this corn. This results in things like high-fructose corn syrup and ethanol fuel.

So for American readers, I need to add in another point. Learn to fastidiously read labels to look for high-fructose corn syrup. You may be horrified to find that most of the foods you enjoy are sweetened with corn syrup. A good option (if your budget allows) is to source from organic specialists like Whole Foods or Trader Joes, who tend to have better quality food available. Eventually, however, you may reach a conclusion which will open up a whole new world of healthy eating – your best option for reducing fructose (and therefore inflammation and AGEs, is to make more of your own food and reduce the amount of packaged food you consume.

One thing to note is that, as we stand now, there is considerable controversy as to exactly which foods either contain the most AGEs or trigger the production of AGEs in the body. For example, some believe butter to be high in a variant of AGEs, whereas others believe we should focus on sugar-related AGEs as being the most dangerous. My position is that, until we get more research in on which foods to avoid, the no-brainer at the moment is to minimize fructose and in particular, avoid high-fructose corn syrup.

At this stage the only supplement with good research backing in terms of reducing the effects of AGEs is the vitamin B1 (thiamine) analog *benfotiamine*. Benfotiamine appears to reduce the damage associated with glycation and inhibits inflammation by modulating a protein known as *nuclear factor-kappaB* (NF-kB).

Identify and treat hypertension (high blood pressure)

It is almost redundant to include this section because throughout this book we are directly dealing with the majority of all the causes of high blood pressure. If you manage stress, reduce alcohol consumption and exercise regularly (all recommended here already), you significantly reduce your chances of developing hypertension.

Probably the only other major point missing from this book is reducing salt intake. The issue of salt intake is complicated because for the majority of the population, salt consumption is not a problem. Salt should really only be targeted when high blood pressure (that hasn't responded to the other dietary and behavioral recommendations) is an issue. For a while there, salt was becoming a kind of "bogeyman" (just like cholesterol was also) and the general population was making wholesale reductions to the amount of salt they consumed. The problem with this is that when you cut out one thing from your diet, you naturally increase another thing (unless you reduce the amount of food you consume, which is unlikely). This meant that broad-based salt reduction was followed by commensurate increases in the consumption of sugar and carbohydrate. That's fine if you have seriously high blood pressure, but not so great for someone with normal to low blood pressure.

Any book on increasing life expectancy must, either directly or indirectly, look at reducing your risk of dying from the major killers. High blood pressure is acknowledged as being one of the main causative factors in preventable death due to heart disease and stroke. The World Health Organization considers high blood pressure to be the number one preventable cause of death worldwide. This is why I need to include a section on high blood pressure. There are many other causes of early mortality that we don't yet have a clear, direct treatment for, such as certain cancers or neurological disease. Whereas with high blood pressure, just some simple lifestyle changes and in certain cases antihypertensive medication, can essentially remove this as a risk factor in your demise.

If you imagine a blocked garden hose turned on for a period of time, bulging in parts, you can also imagine why high blood pressure is such a massive problem. If high blood pressure is left untreated, you are at high risk for something eventually bursting – whether in the heart, brain or elsewhere in the cardiovascular system.

If you haven't already had your blood pressure tested, get it tested immediately. If your blood pressure is found to be on the high side, your doctor will either initially recommend lifestyle changes only, or they may be more cautious and want you to start taking an antihypertensive drug as well. This will particularly be the case if you have dangerously high blood pressure.

The beauty of treating high blood pressure is that it responds well to lifestyle changes and if that isn't enough, the drugs used are also considered relatively safe. The drugs used to treat high blood pressure are possibly the least controversial of all categories of medication. So, whereas we have a massive debate raging on the consequences of statin therapy for "high cholesterol" (inverted commas deliberate), antihypertensive drugs are considered almost universally safe. There are a few different categories, however depending on the doctor and the country you are in, you will most like be prescribed a thiazide diuretic, a calcium channel blocker, an ACE inhibitor or an adrenergic receptor antagonist (beta blockers and alpha blockers).

Don't be afraid to aggressively treat high blood pressure. There are few complications associated with low blood pressure (apart from dizziness-related problems), so it doesn't matter if your treatment overshoots your blood pressure a little to the low side.

However, as mentioned, if you follow the guidelines in this book regarding diet, exercise and stress-reduction, hypertension is unlikely except in cases where there is a strong genetic disposition.

Optimize liver function

As we have seen in the section on glutathione, a healthy liver is central to longevity as it is one of your front line defenses in detoxifying and repairing cellular damage. This organ bears the brunt of the modern lifestyle more than any other organ, as it is the liver that must deal with the consequences of a poor diet and the excess use of various drugs, medicines and alcohol.

Most people are aware of what is required to maintain a healthy heart and brain, however, apart from the general recommendation to "minimize alcohol consumption", the average person would struggle to list any of the other reasons a liver can become dysfunctional or any of the different substances which help to repair it.

Outside of medical circles, almost no-one knows about *N-acetylcysteine and* hardly anyone knows about glutathione.

Ask the average person what the liver actually does, you will generally get either a blank look or a vague statement that *'it processes toxins'* or *'it cleans the blood'*. However, the liver does so much more. For example -

- The liver can create glucose (an important source of energy for your brain in particular) from glycogen, protein and fat

- The liver can create vital amino acids

- The liver creates the majority of all your cholesterol - yes - the amount of cholesterol in your blood is only weakly related to how much you consume via your diet!

- The liver creates triglyceride fats that your body can use for energy

- The liver produces certain substances which enable your blood to coagulate in the event of injury

- In the developing baby, before bone marrow is ready to assume the role, the liver is responsible for producing most of the baby's red blood cells

- The liver synthesizes and processes bile, which your body needs for digesting fats. Bile also facilitates the absorption of vitamin K from the diet. For anyone deficient in vitamin D or currently taking vitamin D supplements to correct a deficiency, vitamin K is incredibly important for ensuring that the body sends dietary calcium to your bones and not to your arteries.

- The liver produces *insulin-like growth factor 1* (IGF-1), a hormone which is hugely important to the natural development of children and continues to have an important role into adulthood.

- The liver breaks down various hormones after they are no longer required

- The liver processes bilirubin, one of the substances responsible for, how should I put this, your poop being brown.

- The liver is responsible for the majority of all drug metabolism. This can be either the processing of toxic substances (such as acetaminophen) or the conversion of a drug taken orally into a metabolite which is active in the body. For example, the popular painkiller codeine itself is virtually inactive; however in the liver, codeine is converted into morphine, a significantly more powerful drug. This is how codeine and similar drugs which require metabolism work.

- The liver converts toxic ammonia into urea via the urea cycle, to enable safe processing of this toxic substance

- The liver also acts as a storage house for a variety of vitamins and minerals including - vitamin A, vitamin D, vitamin B12, vitamin K, iron and copper.

- The liver, supporting the lymphatic system, is responsible for a healthy immune system via the production of various immunity-boosting substances

- The liver produces a hormone involved with regulating healthy blood pressure levels

So what can go wrong?

Hepatitis - this is the most common type of major liver disease, where inflammation of the liver is, except in rare cases, caused by the hepatitis virus.

Alcoholic liver disease - this is the catch-all term for liver diseases such as fatty liver, alcoholic hepatitis and cirrhosis which are all caused by the excess consumption of alcohol. Left untreated, these can lead to liver failure.

What are the symptoms of liver damage or a poorly functioning liver?

- Pale stools - sorry to bring up poop again. Remember bilirubin I just mentioned which gives poop its brown tint? A damaged liver doesn't produce enough of it so pale stools can eventuate

- Dark colored urine

- Jaundice, where the skin or the whites of the eyes can take on a yellow tint. This is because of the poorly functioning liver's inability to correctly process bilirubin, leading to its deposit in the skin

- Abdominal swelling, indigestions, acid reflux and fat-soluble vitamin deficiencies caused by the inability to properly absorb fat

- Fatigue caused by a lack of nutrients and hormones produced by the liver

- Excessive bruising or bleeding due to a lack of that substance I mentioned that enables blood to clot

- A poorly functioning liver can also impact your brain and nervous system, leading to mood changes (particularly depression) and an inability to concentrate.

- Elevated cholesterol levels

If you suspect that you have a poorly functioning liver, before you do anything, visit your doctor and request liver function tests. These tests look for certain enzymes which are associated with the liver. Abnormal levels of these enzymes can point to a potential issue with liver function.

The good news is that the liver has an unequaled ability to regenerate itself. Your liver is an amazing organ which can take most of what life throws at it. Imagine if you cut three-quarters of your finger off and it grew back. This is what the liver is capable of. Under certain circumstances, a person could regrow a new liver from only around a quarter of a normal liver.

This means that, for a person with a healthy diet, who does not take a large amount of legal or illegal drugs (including medicines), who does not consume a large amount of alcohol and who doesn't have any pre-existing genetic or lifestyle related liver disease, you have absolutely no need to be concerned. However, the problem is that many people do drink excessive quantities of alcohol, take illicit drugs, use a variety of medications and follow a poor diet.

The other piece of good news is that the liver responds dramatically to certain supplements. If someone has issues with a poorly functioning liver, through the use of certain supplements, they will see quite dramatic improvements in functioning and reap the consequent longevity-related benefits.

Out of all the various supplements which are promoted for a healthy liver, only four meet my criteria in having solid scientific backing through clinical trials -

- **N-Acetylcysteine (NAC)**

- **Milk thistle (silymarin)**

- **Curcumin**

- **Alpha lipoic acid (ALA)**

Are you starting to see a pattern here?

I have covered NAC, ALA and curcumin in the sections on glutathione and inflammation, so I just need to now cover what is probably the single most powerful liver optimizing supplement available - *milk thistle*.

However I should point out that one of the key ways in which milk thistle heals the liver is the same as the other supplements covered - it increases levels of glutathione.

When I first heard of milk thistle a few years ago, I was initially quite skeptical about claims regarding the ability to detoxify and rejuvenate the liver. Well, I was wrong. Subsequent research uncovered an amazing amount of research on this fascinating herb. The research is unequivocal – milk thistle really does repair the liver.

Milk thistle has been used for 2000 years as natural treatment for various diseases such as kidney, cancer and gall bladder problems, lowering cholesterol levels, hepatitis B and C, spleen disorders, malaria, menstrual problems and swelling of the lungs. It is extracted from the seeds (fruit) of the milk thistle plant and the seeds are used to prepare capsules, extracts, powders, and tinctures. Now, just because something has been used for certain conditions for thousands of years, that doesn't mean that it has been proven to work for those conditions. To prove that something works, you need to conduct randomized, double-blind placebo controlled trials. As I will soon show, it is in these trials that milk thistle has shone.

When we talk about milk thistle as a supplement, in general what we are talking about is a single phenol called *silymarin*, which the milk thistle is high in. If you want to get even more specific, the active constituent of silymarin is called *silibinin (or silibin)*, a flavonoid with powerful antioxidant actions. When you purchase milk thistle as a supplement, in general you are purchasing a standardized extract of silymarin.

Milk thistle has solid evidence backing its use for –

- Repairing liver damage caused by overuse of medications, alcohol and street drugs

- Improving life expectancy for patients with cirrhosis of the liver

- Assisting in the treatment of viral hepatitis

- Preventing acute liver damage from ingesting high doses of hepatotoxic (toxic to the liver) substances such as acetaminophen and Death Cap Mushroom

- Assisting in the treatment of mild depression

- Milk Thistle appears to increase bile solubility, potentially demonstrating benefit in preventing or treating gallstones.

One of the best ways to view milk thistle without getting bogged down in too much detail, is to think of it as a super-potent antioxidant. Milk thistle hunts down free radicals which have been shown to damage cells and accelerate certain aspects of the aging process. Milk Thistle not only acts as an antioxidant itself but also increases the activity of other antioxidants such as *superoxide dismutase*, which we know to be an incredibly powerful fighter of oxidative damage.

However, one of the most interesting aspects of milk thistle is that it has been shown to increase levels of glutathione in the liver by significant amounts, like NAC and ALA.

Milk thistle also acts as an anti-inflammatory by inhibiting levels of *leukotriene*, a pro-inflammatory substance that has been linked to everything from heart disease to cancer to psoriasis.

So, milk thistle repairs the liver, increases glutathione and reduces inflammation. You can see why I initially struggled to work out exactly *where* in this book I should cover this interesting herb.

As you would imagine from a substance that acts as an antioxidant, milk thistle has some solid research backing regarding its anti-cancer properties. Now, whenever I read 'natural therapy' and 'cancer' I immediately get suspicious. Too many times I have heard of a cancer patient refusing chemotherapy to try something like homeopathy, which I strongly oppose. When you are diagnosed with cancer, it is not the time to abandon modern western medicine. However, surprisingly, not only has the anti-cancer action of milk thistle been demonstrated, so has the mechanism by which it acts.

One of the most promising areas of research into a potential cure for cancer has been looking at the blood vessels which feed cancers and thereby allowing them to grow. If you can cut of the blood supply to cancers, you can stop them from spreading. Incredibly, milk thistle has shown to possess exactly this property. Now, let me be clear however – this in no way means that milk thistle can currently be viewed as a viable alternative to pharmaceutical drugs for the treatment of advanced cancers. However, what it does show is a clear mechanism for inhibiting the growth and spread of early cancers. To put it another way, milk thistle could prove to be a useful supplement for those who want to reduce their risk of getting a deadly cancer by stopping early cancers in their tracks. So far, milk thistle has demonstrated the ability to fight prostate, skin, ovarian, colon, breast, lung and cervical cancers.

A 2007 study found that an extract of milk thistle blocked hepatitis C virus (HCV) cell culture infection of human hepatoma cultures. Another study conducted in 2010 found that the eight major compounds that comprise milk thistle, including seven flavonolignans and one flavonoid are all inhibitors of HCV RNA-dependent RNA polymerase.

According to a study published in the journal *Phytotherapy Research* in 2006, milk thistle may also keep insulin levels more stable by regulating or decreasing the blood glucose levels in the body. This is interesting for two reasons – not just the obvious benefits for patients with type 2 diabetes. Insulin is also heavily implicated in weight fain via fat accumulation in the body – particularly around the belly for males. This implies potential uses for milk thistle in the area of weight management. However the evidence at this stage is only preliminary so I wouldn't recommend going out and buying milk thistle to lose weight.

A study also showed that the flavonoid component of milk thistle helped to lower cholesterol and triglyceride levels, which are often high in people who are overweight or obese. High levels of fats in the blood can also lead to increased risk of cardiovascular disease. Triglyceride levels in particular are becoming more and more implicated as one of the key risk factors in heart disease. The ability of fish oil (omega 3 fatty acids) to decrease the risk of heart disease is due in no small part by the ability of fish oil to decrease levels of triglycerides in the blood.

Another case report points to a potential indirect use for milk thistle in the fight against cancer. A woman who was suffering from a type of leukemia was given Milk Thistle extract while being treated with powerful immunosuppressive and steroidal drugs. This patient had required regular treatment breaks due to adverse changes in liver enzyme levels. After treatment with Milk Thistle, the patient's liver enzymes normalized and she was able to continue treatment without further interruption. Naturally this is only a case report, not a clinical trial, however it points to a potential use for milk thistle to maintain a healthy liver when it is being assaulted by potent drugs needed to either cure a cancer patient or extend life expectancy. Fortunately, this potential application for milk thistle has been backed up with a clinical trial.

In this promising double-blind, placebo-controlled trial, a group children who were receiving treatment for acute lymphoblastic leukemia were unfortunately showing signs of hepatotoxicity (liver damage) caused by their chemotherapy drugs. The children were split into two groups with one group receiving milk thistle extract and the other group a placebo. The results of the trial were that the group receiving milk thistle extract showed significantly lower levels of *alanine aminotransferase* than the placebo group. Alanine aminotransferase is a reliable indicator of liver damage, so this result was extremely encouraging and further backed up the previous case report.

Another randomized controlled trial supported by the *National Institute of Diabetes and Digestive and Kidney Diseases* involved patients with hepatitis C who had not responded to antiviral therapy. The study involved assessing all the various herbal medicines and natural therapies to ascertain whether there was any benefit. Out of those taking herbal supplements, over 70% involved milk thistle extract. Patients were surveyed regarding all aspects of their health and wellbeing. The study found that those patients taking milk thistle extract showed significantly fewer adverse symptoms and enjoyed a much higher quality of life. This is extremely encouraging however I should point out that these studies that involve subjects self-reporting are notoriously unreliable. It is very easy to convince yourself that you have better quality of life because you are taking milk thistle – it is much harder to influence levels of alanine aminotransferase by placebo effect alone.

Another report mentions milk thistle as the only effective antidote in patients with liver damage from Death Cap Mushroom (*Amanita Phalloides*) poisoning. Patients received doses of milk thistle extract, which demonstrated clear effectiveness in preventing the liver damage associated with this type of poisoning. Again, the other benefit was that there were no reports of adverse events or side-effects. Naturally, unless you are particularly unlucky, having the antidote for Death Cap Mushroom poisoning has little to do with longevity. However it does give an indication of the potent actions of milk thistle in the body.

However the best kind of clinical trial data comes from meta-analyses, which is where all the results from different trials are put together to create an overall picture of a certain medication or supplement. The two main meta-analyses which have been conducted on Milk Thistle have been a *Cochrane Review* in 2005 and an *Agency for Healthcare Research and Quality* (AHRQ) study. Both of these reviews reached a similar conclusion – that whilst the data on milk thistle for treating diseases of the liver were encouraging, many of the studies were poorly designed and that the actual mechanism by which milk thistle works is still a little unclear. This doesn't mean that they believed milk thistle didn't work, just that it had not yet been proven to the degree to which they would feel comfortable recommending this herb as a front-line treatment for liver diseases.

The Cochrane Review looked at thirteen randomized clinical trials which assessed milk thistle in 915 patients with alcoholic and/or Hepatitis B or C. They concluded that whilst there appeared to be some beneficial effects, there was still a lack of evidence to recommend milk thistle on a widespread basis.

One of the problems with milk thistle, like curcumin, it its low level of bioavailability. What this means is that even though you are taking a potentially large dose, much of it is not absorbed by your body. Recently there has been two fantastic developments in efforts to improve absorption and therefore effectiveness. Firstly, scientists have identified more clearly that silibin is the main active constituent of milk thistle and have subsequently produced purified versions with only silibin. This increases the potency and therefore the ability of the body to absorb enough to obtain the desired benefits. Secondly, a new phospholipid complex call *Siliphos* has been developed. Siliphos is essentially silibin bound with soy-based phospholipids to improve the body's ability to absorb the silibin. This results in dramatically increased levels of silibin in the blood after administration, compared to standard silibin supplementation.

Milk thistle appears to be surprisingly free of any serious adverse effects considering how potently it acts in the body. For some people it can have a mild laxative effect and in massive overdose is can cause nausea, stomach pain, vomiting, headaches, joint pain, indigestion, itching, bloating and diarrhea. However I should point out that you would need to consume a massive dose to see anything like this.

As with just about any supplement, pregnant women should avoid milk thistle as there is no conclusive evidence proving lack of harm (or harm for that matter) at this stage. Any potential liver boosting effects of milk thistle should be put to one side when you are pregnant.

Due to the lack of adverse effects and dangers, there is little requirement for highly specialized or specific dosages, however in general you could target between 400-800mg per day in divided doses.

If you are currently suffering from a diagnosed liver disease such as alcoholic cirrhosis or hepatitis, milk thistle should be an almost automatic option alongside your conventional therapies. As a repairer of your liver, milk thistle is without equal in the herbal world.

However if you are currently relatively healthy but are worried about liver health or put your liver under a lot of strain from alcohol and drugs, I believe you should also make milk thistle one of your front line options for keeping your liver in great condition. People forget that their liver is up there with the heart and brain in terms of importance for your survival. It is involved in so many different functions in the body that that keeping it in the best condition possible should be a priority for anyone looking towards maximizing their own longevity.

Exercise

Exercise is the single greatest thing you can do for your brain. And evolution knows it too, which is why there is a complex system of biochemical reactions that reward you when you exercise.

You have probably heard of the *runner's high* right? You have probably also heard that this "high" comes from endorphins, your body's own internal morphine. Well, it turns out that this is only partly true. But I'll get to that in a bit.

In terms of building a super-brain, the single most important factor is relating to BDNF (*brain-derived neurotrophic factor*), your brain's own "*miracle-gro*" (as I have heard a few other authors refer to it as). BDNF is a protein that helps your existing brain cells to thrive and also helps drive important aspects of neurogenesis – the birth of new neurons. Neurogenesis seems so commonplace nowadays that it is easy to forget that up until only a few years ago it was believed that neurogenesis was impossible. Remember being told that you are born with a certain number of brain cells and can never grow new ones? Well, it turns out that was incorrect.

It also turns out that exercise is the single most powerful behavior you can engage in to stimulate the secretion of BDNF in important parts of the brain such as the hippocampus. The hippocampus is central to a sharp brain (particularly memory recall) and a good mood. The hippocampus of depressed people is often found to have actually shrunk by a measurable amount! The good news is that, of all the areas in your brain, the hippocampus is one of the best at recovering and growing new neurons.

In terms of exercise for neural functioning, there is a great body of work centered on dementia patients, such as those with Alzheimer's. As I often mention, research on Alzheimer's gives us great indications regarding what works to improve cognition and memory.

Therefore, it is unsurprising that multiple studies have shown that exercise improves aspects of dementia both acutely and chronically. What this means is that a single episode of exercise (say, jogging for 30 minutes) increases production of BDNF and improves markers of cognition (acutely), while a continued exercise program gives additional benefits which gradually accumulate (chronically).

However it is in the area of depression and anxiety treatment that exercise has the most research behind it.

In his book Spark!: How exercise will improve the performance of your brain, John Ratey cites study after study which clearly demonstrates the link between exercise and not only mood, but cognitive function also. If you are serious about understanding the nexus between exercise and brain health, I strongly urge you to read books such as Ratey's. He was trying to get the message out about this important topic before anyone else – a true trailblazer.

As I mentioned in the introduction to this section, for quite a few years now the accepted wisdom was that runner's high was caused by endorphins. In fact, it's hard to believe that only a few years before that, we still had no idea about the existence of your body's own internal "morphine". For years scientists wondered why exactly was it that your brain had its own locks (opiate receptors) which morphine and other opiates (the keys) perfectly fit. Eventually endorphins (literally "endogenous morphine") were discovered as being the natural painkilling chemical produced by your body in times of stress or physical pain.

So that perfectly explains why you feel good when you exercise and why exercise treats depression right? As with anything to do with the brain, it is a little more complicated.

There is a drug called *naloxone* which completely neutralizes the effects of opiates on the brain. If you take naloxone and then shoot heroin, you don't get high. Which is why it is often a component of addiction treatment. It turns out that if you give someone naloxone and then they exercise, the naloxone only negates some aspects of the mood boost you get from exercise.

Subsequent research on both animals and humans has shown that exercise also increases levels of your *monoamines* – serotonin, dopamine and norepinephrine. Yes, exercising really is like popping a happy pill.

Exercise also improves oxygenation of the brain through improved blood flow. Your brain is a massive oxygen and energy sponge, so anything which improves delivery of this vital fuel to where it's needed is going to be hugely beneficial.

Finally, exercise also helps in an indirect way by improving one of the most important aspects of brain health – sleep. Sleep is where your brain does the majority of its repair work – particularly during *slow wave sleep* (stage 3 & 4 "NREM" sleep) which is your deepest stage of sleep.

As you probably know, while you are asleep, your brain goes through various stages which can all be measured with a polysomnograph. You are probably most familiar with one of these stages – REM ("rapid eye movement") sleep. Slow wave sleep is when the majority of your brain's repair work happens. Exercise increases slow wave sleep, meaning that not only do you wake more refreshed than you would otherwise be, but your brain has been able to accelerate its repair work.

There is still some debate as to why exercise helps with sleep quality and quantity. I believe that it is a combination of factors. Firstly, exercise burns off a lot of stress hormones and neurotransmitters such as cortisol and norepinephrine, leading to increased relaxation and deeper sleep – you sleep much more lightly when you are stressed or physiologically aroused. Secondly, exercise, when done in the late afternoon particularly, artificially raises your core body temperature. Scientists still aren't sure why, but raising your body temperature a few hours before bed will increase slow wave sleep. This is the reason why hot baths before bed also increase slow wave sleep. The cooling that happens as your body slides down into sleep, appears to set off some kind of biochemical reaction that leads to better sleep quality.

So, if we acknowledge that exercise super-charges your brain and improves your mood, the next question is – *What kind of exercise?*

My philosophy is always to focus on doing what you enjoy. If you force yourself to do something you hate, you will soon give up and be back at square one. If you hate jogging, don't try to force yourself to jog. Be guided by how you feel. After reading so often about how jogging before breakfast accelerates weight loss, I decided to force myself to jog as soon as I woke up. It only took me a few times before I realized I hated it so much that I would never keep it up. However, come 11am each morning, I love nothing better than to hit the gym or even go for the occasional run.

Ideally you will be doing a mixture of – cardiovascular exercise, strength training and stretches. I am a massive fan of H.I.I.T (*high intensity interval training*) for brain health. I am also a busy, impatient guy, so I love to get my exercise done quickly. So don't think that you need to spend an hour on a treadmill. You could literally find a grassed area and do, say, 5 x 100 meter sprints and you would see massive benefits for your brain. It could be all over in 10 minutes. There is a whole new science emerging recently which supports the idea that the best kind of exercise is short in duration and high intensity.

Pick what you love and just keep at it. Remember, one of the mainstays of depression treatment is walking. Yes, just getting out of the house and walking at a leisurely pace can have a dramatic effect on symptoms of depression.

Get socially connected

We humans are social animals. We have evolved to form deep bonds with a community of friends and family around us. Some evolutionary psychologists have even hypothesized that the reason we needed to develop such a complex and powerful brain (in my case this is debatable) was to manage a complex web of co-operative relationships with those around us.

One of the easiest ways to see this is to consider what happens when people become isolated. In general, if we are separated from loved ones or even from any human being at all, we become depressed and occasionally our grasp on reality can even unravel.

In his landmark book "The Blue Zones: Lessons for Living Longer from people who lived the longest", author Dan Buettner identified certain locations around the world that are characterised by an unusually high number of centenarians. They were - Okinawa (Japan), Sardinia (Italy), Nicoya (Costa Rica), Icaria (Greece) and a group of Seventh Day Adventists in Loma Linda, California.

After identifying these longevity superstars, the most important point should be identifying why these populations live longer and healthier lives. Each of these areas had their own unique tendencies which were believed to be contributing factors. So for example, the Loma Linda Seventh Day Adventists ate plenty of nuts, whereas the Sardinians drank polyphenol-rich red wine.

Where this line of inquiry got really interesting however, was when researchers looked for unifying factors that held consistent across all of these "blue zones". In the below Venn diagram you can see that these common traits were - emphasis on family, no smoking, regular physical activity, social engagement and the consumption of legumes.

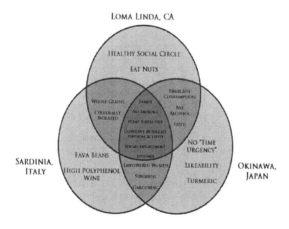

(Chart source: Wikipedia)

I have to admit being surprised to see legumes in there, considering the range of nutritional shortcomings they have. My first instinct is to think that legumes are there mainly by chance - I think it is correlation not causation. However I am also prepared to accept the possibility that there is something as yet unidentified regarding the health benefits of legumes. One thing is for certain however - legumes are not sending these people to an early grave, so perhaps we need to do more study into this vegetarian staple.

So, the thing that immediately sticks out is the fact that two of the unifying factors in the blue zones are "family" and "social engagement", which I would argue are one and the same in terms of coming under the general umbrella of *socialization promoting longevity*.

As I have spent an improbably large amount of time recently researching longevity and the factors that promote it, the importance of maintaining social connections is the single, unchanging factor. Some groups that are long lived eat plenty of fish, while others are mainly vegetarian. Some drink no alcohol, whereas others drink red wine. However all of them maintain a rich network of social and familial ties. Or to put it another way, when different groups are studied, no one ever cites "isolation and loneliness" as a factor in their longevity.

To learn the importance of social ties for a person's longevity, it is helpful to look at what goes wrong in your brain and body when you are isolated.

Fortunately, in the area of neuroscience and mental health, there is a large body of work we can draw from when looking at the brain of a lonely, isolated person. Isolation is a potent trigger for mood disorders, leading to various changes in the brain and cardiovascular system.

Study into the effects of isolation on the human mind can be traced back to renowned psychotherapist Frieda Fromm-Reichmann. Reichmann's seminal 1959 work *"On Loneliness"* is considered the starting point of modern-day loneliness studies. This has led to a variety of studies into the neurobiological effect of isolation and loneliness. One particular study showed that a lack of social interaction as a young animal (whether a human or a rodent) had enduring negative effects on the human brain such as dysfunctional myelin sheaths (the fatty tubes that protect the axon component of a neuron). Functional myelin are vital for normal nerve transmission, as we can see from the progressive neurological disease multiple sclerosis, which is caused by auto-immune medicated destruction of myelin.

Also, isolation leads to chronically lowered levels of the feel-good neurotransmitter serotonin. It is one of the bizarre ironies of major depression that being depressed causes people to withdraw from the most powerful antidepressant known - rich and varied social contact. However therein lies a rich lesson also - in some cases one of the quickest and most effective ways to reverse depression is to socialize.

Isolation appears to be particularly lethal for the elderly, accelerating the rate at which cognition and memory declines. And this is not just rare occurrences either. A 2010 survey in the US found that more than a third of elderly people consider themselves to be "chronically lonely". Any broad-based effort by government to promote longevity or the health of the elderly, must, by definition, pay particular attention to alleviating this chronic loneliness. There are many things we can do as a society to ensure that the elderly don't live out their days in a level of isolation that is hastening their demise. Perhaps we can redirect certain community service activities away from picking up rubbish or cleaning graffiti off walls and back towards spending quality time with the elderly.

One thing we must be careful of, however, is to avoid applying blanket generalizations to what is a diverse group of people on the planet. We must refrain from defining loneliness purely in terms of physical isolation from other human beings. It is possible for certain people to spend their life at various cocktail parties and shindigs, yet feel interminably lonely. There must be a connection between the person and the environment. If you forced a shy, socially anxious person to spend their life at dinner parties, you would possibly be harming them, not helping. Not only do we need to differentiate between natural extroverts and natural introverts, we need to differentiate between someone who is an introvert and someone who is pathologically shy. As Susan Cain points out in her brilliant book Quiet: The power of introverts in a world that can't stop talking, there is a difference between the two and the key word is "pathological". Being an introvert is not necessarily pathological, whereas being painfully shy is.

So whether you are applying this concept for yourself or whether we are looking at broad measures to increase longevity via social interaction, we need to account for variations in personality. This is extremely challenging however. If you are reading this now and you tend to be introverted, do you have a clear idea whether forcing yourself to socialize would be beneficial or not? My advice would be that if you are depressed and alone, you have nothing to lose by forcing yourself to socialize. If for some reason you find it distressing and believe it may be exacerbating your condition, then by all means stop. However I tend to believe that genuine introverts who thrive in isolation are exceedingly rare. By nature, I tend to isolate myself and withdraw into my own little world. However, when I spend certain periods doing a lot of socialization, it does give a noticeable mood boost. I am not particularly beset by bad moods often, however I have noticed on many occasions I was in a bad mood and was dreading an upcoming social engagement (slightly lowered serotonin driving my urge to withdraw?), yet when I started talking to people at the party (or whatever it was) my mood would noticeably brighten in quite dramatic fashion.

You are fighting a lot of evolutionary force by isolating yourself. Evolution (if you could give it humanoid desires) really, really wants you to socialize. Humans are relatively weak if you compare us to the other predators that were prowling the African savannah. What has set us apart throughout history has been our ability to co-operate. Whether we are co-operating to bring down a large prey animal, building huts, protecting the tribe or raising children, it has been this factor which most evolutionary biologists cite as a key difference between man and even our nearest primate relatives.

Throughout human evolution, isolating yourself has not been a good idea at all. You were likely to either starve or be eaten in short order. So your biology sends you strong messages to create multitudinous co-operative and emotional connections with other humans. Just like your brain gives you liberal spurts of dopamine to reward you for finding high-calorie food or a potential mate, your brain sends you a strong message as if to say *Hey you. Get out there and make connections with people. I am withholding all this sweet, sweet serotonin until you do so.*

One thing we need to take into consideration however, is that a lack of social contact possibly makes us feel bad because of conditioned connotations as well. Society can generalize loneliness or isolation as being "sad" - hence the expression "sad & lonely". So are we sad because isolation is inherently depressing or because we are conditioned to think it is so? I tend to still think there is something neurobiological at work, because of what we have seen with rodent tests. Rodents are not brought up to think that "alone" should equal "sad".

However, if we look to meditative contemplatives we can see that with extensive training, sometimes this reaction can be retrained. Over the last few thousand years, Buddhist monks, Indian yogis and other adepts of contemplative traditions have institutionalized the practice of spending large chunks of time in complete isolation. Tibetan lamas, for example, have a tradition of retiring to a cave somewhere for months of meditation with no human contact.

While beginners who try extended period of secluded meditation can risk triggering psychosis or other mental illness, advanced meditators emerge from these periods enveloped in a kind of supernatural bliss. So why are these select few able to run counter to our understanding of socialization's effects on mood and longevity? Extended periods of isolation are characterized by an intense awareness of both the internal world and each word of what must seem like an endless monologue. Perhaps their practice of mindfulness allows them to take the emotional sting out of this incessant chatter? I don't know for sure, however it points to an interesting area of future research because, if we can identify exactly what is the difference between these people and ourselves, we may be able to create targeted future therapies.

I imagine that there are various evolutionary reasons why face to face socializing is more effective, however you also need to be pragmatic. Perhaps you are particularly socially anxious or live in an isolated part of the world. Use the internet to connect, whether through dating sites, social networks or gaming communities. Each time you type something and something comes back from another human, that's a connection.

Also, it could be of use to practice mindfulness, emulating our meditative contemplatives. Mindfulness therapy for mood disorders is one of the fastest growing sub-types of modern-day cognitive behavioral therapy. By practicing mindfulness, perhaps you are able to mitigate isolation as a possible causative factor in a shortened life-span.

However, at the end of the day, the beauty of socialization as a longevity-enhancing strategy is that your single act of connecting with someone socially has the ability to set off a beneficial chain reaction. The most obvious example is our previous example of someone keeping a lonely elderly person company. This act creates two "longevity units" (a completely made-up word by the way) concurrently. Your longevity is enhanced by both the social connection and the self-esteem boost you will get from doing something seemingly altruistic. The elderly person's longevity is also increased by a certain number of "longevity units" (you could argue that they get more units because at their age they would expect to get more noticeable benefit from social connections).

Where this gets truly interesting is where your increased socialization sets off a chain reaction. If we acknowledge that happier people socialize more (both as cause and effect, it goes both ways), then surely there is the likelihood that your act leads to other people socializing more as well. It has the potential to go on endlessly.

All the antioxidants in the world won't offset the life-span shortening effects of isolation. It needs to be a priority.

Reduce stress

If I told you that stress will send you to an early grave, it wouldn't be particularly surprising right? What about if I also told you that stress would also help you to live longer? Surely they can't both be correct can they?

The key is to specify the type of stress. There is a beneficial type called *eu*stress and the more pernicious type known as *di*stress. Eustress is the occasional stressful event that pushes you to achieve a goal or overcome a challenge. This is the kind of stress for which you are evolutionarily prepared - stressful event followed by action, followed by resolution. Distress is the problem. When we refer to stress, we are usually referring to distress.

Your body is singularly unprepared for the type of chronic, unrelenting stress that often typifies modern life. Think about the tyrant boss, for example. Your brain and endocrine system has no correlate from which to draw from in order to deal effectively with this kind of stress.

It is for this reason that stress is such a noxious aspect of modern life, hastening the demise of far too many people. If we just look at cardiovascular related deaths alone and consider the proportion of those where high blood pressure was a causative factor, and consider the role that stress plays in high blood pressure (hypertension), stress must be considered one of the major causes of premature death.

Chronic stress is ruinous for the human body and brain. One of the main problems is the chronically elevated levels of the glucocorticoid hormone *cortisol* that stress causes. Cortisol is hugely important for many functions. Cortisol helps you wake up each morning (it waxes and wanes appropriately in sympathy with your circadian rhythm) and helps you to deal with acutely stressful events. The problems start to occur when stress is unrelenting and cortisol remains elevated for long periods of time.

Cortisol is particularly toxic for your hippocampus, the part of your brain responsible for a range of functions linked to memory recall and context detection. Even in a test tube, cortisol damages hippocampal neurons. It is therefore unsurprising that chronic stress is a known causative factor in dementia, where years of elevated cortisol has gradually impaired the hippocampus.

However the damage is not just isolated to the brain and cardiovascular system. Chronically elevated cortisol is responsible for, or implicated in, a litany of health problems including - insulin resistance, impaired immune system, type 2 diabetes, fat around the belly (in men), decreased bone density and libido problems.

The solution, however, is not to lock yourself in a padded room to avoid any possible source of stress. As I mentioned a moment ago, certain types of acute stress are actually good for you as they help you achieve goals or avoid danger.

Regular but brief stressful episodes are also important as they make you stronger via the process of *hormesis*. In biology, hormesis refers to a small dose of something conferring consequent increased levels of resistance to that particular stressor. In one sense, this is just a fancy was of saying - *what doesn't kill you will make you stronger*. The most common example of this is a vaccine, where you get a small, survivable dose of something infectious or dangerous and are then immune to it from that point on.

So please don't create a form of chronic stress by worrying about occasional acute stress. That occasional stress of the upcoming presentation or the final exam is good for you in most cases.

However, there are a few complicating factors.

Firstly, each of us has a different reaction to stress. Stress is cumulative. When researchers have studied cases of major depression they found something interesting. In a large number of cases, there was a gradual accumulation of stressful experiences which then reached a tipping point where something then *broke* inside the person in question. They lost their job, their spouse left them, one of their parents died and then suddenly something snaps and major depression eventuates.

The interesting thing is that some people snap at a certain point, others snap at another point and another group doesn't snap no matter how much stress is heaped on. The only thing people have to go on is there genetic heritage. If you have a depressive parent or one that went through a breakdown of some sort, you clearly have to exercise particular caution in how much stress you allow to permeate your world.

The other problem is that the relationship between stimuli (the stress) and the reaction (a breakdown or depressive episode) is not linear. It is like a dropped coffee cup. If you drop a coffee cup from a small distance above the ground it won't break. Then you raise it up a little higher - it still doesn't break. As you gradually raise the cup up higher, at a certain tipping point if you drop the cup it will shatter. It's not as if each time you drop it, the cup gets a little bit damaged. The stress (hitting the ground) and the relationship to the reaction (the cup breaking) is not linear. At a certain point it goes from "not broken" to "broken". This analogy is helpful because it is easy to visualize but it is not entirely accurate. For this analogy to be accurate in terms of its application to stress, each time you drop the cup you are actually making it a little stronger. The problem is - who knows at what height the cup will suddenly shatter if dropped?

Similarly with chronic stress, in terms of the brain, we see that at a certain point something snaps inside the person and mental illness results. Here is where the cup analogy shines however. If you were to glue the cup back together so all the pieces fit perfectly, now when you drop the cup it shatters from a much lower height. The correlate for this is the unfortunate fact that an episode of major depression makes you susceptible to further episodes.

Major depression is closer to a heart attack in the sense that once it happens, you are dramatically more vulnerable to it happening again. A heart attack doesn't make the heart muscle stronger, whereas the micro-tears on your skeletal muscles that you get from weight training, *do* actually make those muscles stronger. So for most people, occasional bouts of acute stress is like lifting weights. There is a small, survivable shock that makes the *whole* stronger.

However chronic stress is an entire beast altogether. Keep in mind that I have only really addressed one effect of chronic stress (major depression), however as I mentioned earlier there are a raft of other consequences to keep in mind. It would be a mistake to read this and think *Well, I don't have any mental illness in my family and I am able to take all the stress life is able to throw at me.* How about that grandfather that had lifelong hypertension and died early of a heart attack? What about the aunt who developed type 2 diabetes? That breaking point within every person is different. The weakest link in all of us goes first. What is your own weakest link that would be vulnerable to stress? For some people, they develop insomnia. For others, they need to drink alcohol to cope.

When they learn about eustress and distress, many people struggle to discern which is which, as the line between them can become blurred.

Two of the keys are - *control* and a *sense of purpose.*

One of the classic (and cruel - everyone should take a moment to thank animals that suffer for our benefit) experiments done on mice involves subjecting them to electric shocks at random intervals. What researchers find is that if the mice have a degree of control over their environment (such as an ability to quickly escape to a safe zone when the floor becomes electrified), they appear to maintain a relatively unchanged disposition. However, if the shocks come randomly and the mice have no way of escaping, very soon they start manifesting various biomarkers of depression or an anxiety disorder. The difference is control.

A similar mammalian correlate is the difference between an alpha male and a subordinate male in a group of primates. The poor downtrodden monkeys have markedly lower levels of serotonin than the alphas. They are at the mercy of another animal, with no control over their environment.

The human correlate is someone harassed by a despotic boss at work or someone who is dominated by an abusive partner. There is a reason why CEOs often strut around their domain with a pleasant disposition (apart from the fact that that are almost guaranteed to be an extrovert) - their neurobiological status is completely different to the office gopher on the bottom rung of the company ladder.

Likewise, a common trigger for depression in humans is a feeling that their situation is hopeless, beyond their control to ameliorate. Uncontrolled stress is therefore, unsurprisingly, an extremely common trigger for a nervous breakdown (which is really just an outdated expression for major depression) - because it features two potent breakdown triggers - stress and a lack of control.

Let's glance again at the evolutionary forces which underpin so much of our behavior and biology. What happens when an animal is trapped or cornered? Its body is flooded with the biomarkers of its fight or flight system - cortisol, noradrenaline, glucose and various inflammatory substances such as cytokines (in case you need to repair damage from a wound sustained in defending yourself).

Naturally, you can't just magically turn into a CEO, however there are other ways of achieving the same result. As you would imagine, your first task is to work out whether you can indeed just remove yourself (the "flight" in "fight or flight") from whatever it is that possibly makes you feel trapped. Sometimes people have a mental block and believe their situation is inescapable when in fact it is. Often it is possible to leave that abusive partner. Sometimes it is possible to quit your job and change to something less distressing. Here is where the real magic happens. Sometimes just realizing you can escape a situation reduces the stress associated with it. This is because part of the stress is due to the situation itself and part of the stress is due to your perception of it as being inescapable.

However if you can't escape your current situation due to whatever reason, you must then work to reframe it. Let's use weights training as an example. If you are someone who lifts weights at the gym, you are voluntarily subjecting yourself to often intense pain as you push yourself. However, if you were subjected to this same degree of pain each day due to a physical ailment, your stress reaction would be completely different. So the key is not the pain itself but the context under which it arises.

The key is to have a sense of purpose. If you don't even want to escape a situation, it will be significantly less stressful, and even the stress that does remain will not have the same deleterious effects on your health.

An eleven year study of elderly people by the NIH in the US found that those who had a strong sense of purpose lived longer and happier lives than those who didn't. Injecting purpose into a stressful life can be the difference between living past 100 and dying of a sudden heart attack in mid-life. More on sense of purpose later in the book.

Don't accept eustress as unavoidable. Do something about it.

Understand the impact of risky behavior on your life-expectancy

To again use an extreme to illustrate a point, there is no point following every principle mentioned in this book while you spend your weekends base-jumping and driving your car at injudiciously high speeds. If you want to live to 100 and beyond, you need to address not just biological aging, but behavior that exposes your life to risk.

Now for some, the idea of giving up their adrenaline-charged extreme sports sounds like their own personal idea of hell. That's fine. As long as you have a clear idea in your mind of the risks you are exposing yourself to and you are happy with the odds. Depression will also kill you before your time, so clearly you need to do the stuff that makes you happy, dangerous or not.

But remember that risk is cumulative and additive. Let me give the example of driving and skydiving. Skydiving proponents love to defend the safety of the sport (which I admit is much safer than you would imagine). A website I found has arrived at the odds of dying in a parachuting accident as 1 in 100,000 (1 death for every 100,000 jumps), whereas the chance of dying in a motor vehicle accident in any given year is stated as being 1 in 6000.

The first problem with this is where you have multiple jumps each year, as any but the most casual of skydivers would have. Each jump incrementally increases your chances of dying. Each time you repeat a risky activity, you are exposing yourself to additive risk. So if you occasionally speed while driving, it is much less risky than someone who habitually speeds.

The second problem I have with this logic is that it employs a fallacy of logic by comparing driving your car to skydiving. Driving your car is, for many people, an unavoidable part of life. They need to commute to work or to be able to get around and do their shopping. By skydiving (or a similar activity with inherent risk), you are *adding* to the base risk of driving. Unless someone never drives in a car, this comparison is pointless in terms of assessing the relative risk of each activity.

Now I don't mean to pick on skydiving, which actually is a surprisingly safe sport. Many sports have a higher perceived level of risk because the risks are so visible. Skydiving (1 in 100,000 risk) and bungee jumping (1 in 500,000 risk) appear risky because the means of your demise is so readily apparent. In actual fact the riskiest activities are often the ones associated with unlikely means of demise. So before you engage in an activity (either on a regular basis or as a one-off), make sure you have assessed the risks in a logical way.

Remember, the key word is *additive*. Each risk doesn't occur in a vacuum. To give an extreme example, say you ride a motorcycle without a helmet, smoke a pack of cigarettes each day, regularly go base jumping (and yes, I think it would be exceedingly unlikely for someone who smokes a pack a day of cigarettes to go base jumping - this is just for example's sake), drive well over the speed limit, abuse recreational drugs, never exercise and enjoy scuba diving just off Seal Island in South Africa. How likely do you think it would be for you to reach 100? So while the individual risk of an activity is low, the risks increase exponentially each time you repeat the activity and there is also additive risk for each additional other risky activity you engage in.

Here are some of the most common ways to reduce your life expectancy by additive risk -

Use a motorcycle as your main means of transportation. Adding "no helmet" to this puts you in the shallow end of the gene pool.

Smoke cigarettes. Goes without saying right? Here are a couple of damning statistics in case you needed convincing. Lifelong smoking reduces your life expectancy by 25 YEARS. Each packet of cigarettes you smoke, takes 28 minutes off your life. However it is pointless to even mention cigarettes because if you are reading a book on living to 100 and beyond, you are highly unlikely to be a smoker.

Abuse recreational drugs. Each drugs has its own particular risk. For example, heroin is surprisingly non-toxic for the human body (cue hysterical "just say no" people picketing my house). If you were to take oral heroin in controlled dosages, the worst you risk (in terms of damage to the body) is chronic constipation and some relatively benign immune-system issues. The problem with heroin is the dose escalation required to mitigate tolerance and the lack of QC processes wherever the heroin is produced, leading to inconsistent potency and therefore risk of overdose. Not to mention the additive risk of HIV or hepatitis from sharing needles. The contrasts with other drugs like inhalants or methamphetamine (meth), which destroy your body and brain in quick order. If you insist on smoking marijuana, seek out older strains and avoid the newer super-potent strains. Marijuana traditionally had a balanced proportion of *Tetrahydrocannabinol* (which is pro-psychotic) and *cannabidiol* (anti-psychotic). Newer strains have had the cannabidiol bred out, which some researchers believe is the reason why there is such a big problem with marijuana triggering psychotic disorders. If you or your family have any history of schizophrenia, please avoid marijuana altogether.

Drink alcohol in any quantity of 250ml per day. According to the National Cancer Institute, alcohol consumption increases your risk for a range of cancers - particularly cancers of the head or neck, liver, esophagus and breast. If you just read this and you enjoy alcohol, have a quick think about what was the first thought that came into your head when you read this. People are often happy to do anything in books such as these except give up alcohol. Take a moment to ponder what this potentially means regarding your relationship with alcohol. Alcohol is a potent toxin for the body that has just happened to become a social norm. If alcohol was discovered today it would be immediately made illegal. Sorry to sound like a wowser, however it is my responsibility to illuminate all risks. It is then up to you to decide whether you are comfortable with your odds.

These are just a couple of examples. It is up to you to make a clear assessment of the activities you engage in that add to your risk of early death. Perhaps you enjoy jumping into the wild animal enclosures at zoos or something else I have no ability to imagine.

Assess these activities and then make an informed decision as to whether you want to continue. There is nothing wrong with engaging in risky activities that give you a love for life. Just understand the risks involved so you are not taken by surprise when you find yourself walking through a dark tunnel with your dead grandma waiting for you on the other side.

Healthy diet

The problem with dietary recommendations is that the science is constantly evolving. Remember all those years you were told to avoid eggs because they gave you high cholesterol and increased your risk of heart disease? Now eggs are recognized as one of nature's super-foods, with just about every vitamin you need. If I was trapped on a desert island with only one choice of food, eggs would be near the top *(and yes, I realize that I could possibly just order "Asian beef stir fry" or some other complete meal, if I was particularly clever).*

Similarly, we are in the midst of a major shift in our understanding of nutrition. While there are some nutritionists who are still behind the times and some doctors who disagree, we are seeing the following general trends in nutrition -

- Saturated fat does not "clog your arteries" and is in fact vital for a range of biochemical processes. The villain is in fact trans-fatty acids and polyunsaturated vegetable oils (such as soybean or canola oil). If you are still using margarine instead of (heavenly) butter, you may want to do a little research. If you are still worried about butter, at least switch to spreads made from olive oil.

- Olive oil - speaking of olive oil, it remains the one single fat that everyone agrees is healthy. Some people still believe butter is unhealthy, whereas olive oil remains untouched by controversy.

- Vegetables - and speaking of controversy, vegetables are still the main category of food that everyone agrees is good for you. Particularly leafy greens such as broccoli.

- Whole grains (or any grain-based products) are not particularly healthy. Adding roughage to grain does not miraculously make it healthy if you are eating plenty of fiber-rich vegetables. However there are a few exceptions where there is still healthy debate and ongoing research. For example, rice appears to be a more healthy option than wheat-based products such as bread (Some scientists think this is because rice has a lot of the bad stuff leeched out when it is boiled)

- Legumes - Legumes (such as soy) have vocal supporters and opponents on both sides. Legumes contain some healthy phytochemicals and some not so healthy ones. Do your own research and make up your mind. I tend to think that a few beans here and there don't do me any particular harm. If in doubt, stick to vegetables.

- Avoid quick-digesting carbohydrates such as bread, pasta, rice and potatoes if you want to lose weight.

- Animal protein is good for you and can promote weight loss. This point used to drive opponents of the Atkins weight loss method crazy. They would invent all kinds of explanations why people would lose dramatic amounts of weight eating mainly fat and protein. I have seen similar experiences first hand - people struggling to lose any weight by going "low fat", then switching to Paleo or Atkins-style diets and losing a heap of weight.

- Calories in, calories out - Speaking of losing weight eating animal protein and fat, if someone tries to tell you that weight loss is just a question of "calories in, calories out" tell them that "the 1980s called and they want their weight loss suggestions back". This advice completely ignores the important aspect regarding the hormones that control hunger and what your body does with the energy it consumes. Still skeptical? Tomorrow morning, eat a large serving of white bread. Then, record what time you subsequently become hungry again and the intensity of your hunger. The next morning, eat only animal protein such as meat or egg (try to match the actual calories as closely as possible - you may have to weigh your food). Then measure when you became hungry and how hungry you were. OK, back now? Pretty amazing wasn't it? Eating carbohydrates makes you hungry due to the insulemic response. Eating animal protein keeps you fuller for longer. Remember those morbidly obese people you saw on television who you thought might be just lazy or lacking willpower? It turns out that most of these people have a certain hormonal status (mainly focusing on ghrelin, leptin and insulin) that causes them to rarely feel full and be almost constantly hungry. They are often in a state of perpetual torture. This shows the power of your hormones to control hunger and fat storage. Remember this next time someone tells you that it's all about "calories in, calories out".

- Fruit juice is not healthy - An apple is healthy. A glass of apple juice made from 5-10 apples is not healthy in the slightest. From an evolutionary perspective, your body has no way of processing such a massive blast of sugar as you get from a glass of juice such as apple or orange juice. A glass of juice wreaks havoc on your blood sugar levels and insulin response. Everyone knows that soda is unhealthy, but many people still think that fruit juice is a healthy alternative. It isn't. Stick to water for thirst and if you feel like fruit, eat fruit, not fruit juice.

- Eating a high-fat or high-cholesterol diet gives you heart disease - Tell this to the ethnic groups such as the *Maasai* and the *Inuit* who consume almost entirely animal fat and protein yet experience much less heart disease than westerners. Dietary cholesterol consumption is not only a poor predictor of heart disease but also a poor predictor of serum cholesterol levels! That's right - the majority of your cholesterol level is determined by genetics and liver function, not the amount of cholesterol you consume. One of the greatest scandals in nutrition over the past 50 years has been the lipid hypothesis, which hypothesized that your level of fat consumption determines your risk of heart disease. The frustrating thing was that you are now told to avoid fatty foods because of two dubious events -

    o Ancel Keys' *Seven Countries Study* - this was the first study published that showed a link between fat consumption and heart disease. There's just one problem. There were actually 22 countries' data available and Keys cherry picked the countries that fit his hypothesis. He excluded countries (such as the Netherlands and Norway) where there was a high-fat diet but less heart disease, and countries that consume less fat but have higher heart disease (like Chile).

o The USDA - Keys' work was picked up by the USDA (whose main function is to promote US grain-based agriculture) and used to promote a grain-based diet. Have a look at the USDA food pyramid -

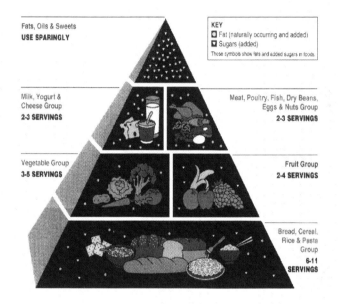

(Chart source - Wikipedia)

Notice anything odd? Yep - all the foods on the bottom are made from the grains that the USDA promotes. Don't you think it is strange that bread would be on the bottom below vegetables?

- Seafood - Another type of food that is almost free from controversy (similarly to vegetables and olive oil) is seafood - particularly fatty fish that are rich in Omega 3 fatty acids. If you remain nervous about saturated fat and animal protein, a diet focused around seafood and vegetables is a risk-free option. Just avoid fish at the top of the food chain (such as tuna, shark, and swordfish) which can be high in mercury.

- Avoid processed meat - While there is nothing wrong with animal protein, you should avoid processed meat (smoked, cured or in any way processed) which is associated with increased risk of certain cancers such as bowel cancer. Each new study that comes out reinforces this association, including a huge analysis in Europe that looked at more than 400,000 people. No-one knows for sure why this is the case. Some researchers think it is because processed meats (like bacon) are often consumed by people who are not focused on a healthy diet. This is the reason why vegetarian diets are sometimes associated with longer life-expectancy - the average person eating a vegetarian diet is more likely to be concerned about their health and make healthier lifestyle choices. Other researchers think that the problem with processed meats may be their nitrate content. Whatever the reason, there is enough evidence for you to avoid processed meat where possible *(Note - hypocrisy warning - the author wishes to disclose that he has a love affair with bacon and, try as he may, he cannot break the hold that this delicious variety of processed meat has on him)*

So, based on the current science and the information we have, the following foods should form a major part of your diet -

- Leafy green vegetables such as broccoli or Chinese cabbage (*bok choy*) - This is as close as you get to the perfect food source

- Seafood - With particular focus on foods rich in omega 3 such as salmon and sardines. Oysters (farmed in areas free of pollution) are a great natural source of zinc.

- Fruit (particularly berries) - Just about every type of fruit has unique selling points. Bananas are packed full of potassium and apples are packed full of a healthy type of fiber called pectin. However the undisputed champions (especially in terms of anti-aging benefits) are berries, which, as previously mentioned, are full of various polyphenols that fight oxidative stress. Plus, berries are relatively lower in fructose.

- If you are going to eat red meat, ensure it is grass-fed (not grain-fed). Grain-fed meat is high in omega 6, whereas grass-fed meat is high in omega 3.

Anti-aging supplements

This tends to be the area that people instinctively get initially attracted to whenever they want to delay the process of aging. There is something seductive and appealing about taking a pill that does all the hard work and you can sit back and reap the rewards. Unfortunately no such pill exists. If it did, everybody would be taking it and you would know its name.

Likewise, no pill is ever going to fully offset poor lifestyle choices. If you spend your life on the couch eating garbage, no pill is going to save you. Anti-aging supplements should be viewed as the last 5%. They are not going to do the heavy-lifting in terms of getting you to 100 and beyond, however they can help prevent certain diseases or aging processes that have the ability to strike you down ahead of time.

Anti-aging supplements can also be quite expensive, so if you can't afford them, don't worry - there are many ways in which you can more than make up for their effects. For example, N-acetylcysteine increases levels of glutathione, but so too does exercise. Curcumin increases levels of BDNF, but again, so too does exercise.

Here are some of the supplements with the strongest research backing in terms of their ability to delay or reverse the biological signs of aging. Note that I have only included substances with either proven efficacy or safety. For example, there are many proponents of hormone injections such as DHEA or human growth hormone, however the safety of this practice is not demonstrated yet. Indeed many categorically believe that these kinds of hormone injects are not safe. Similarly, the anti-rejection drug (it stops organ rejection - it doesn't stop someone denying your entreaties for affection) *sirolimus* (*rapamycin*) has shown a promising ability to increase the life-span of mice, however this is also just at the research stage.

Resveratrol - As mentioned earlier, exhibits the ability to increase longevity in mice by mimicking the effects of caloric restriction

CoQ10 - Promotes mitochondrial function and cardiac health.

Curcumin - Reduces inflammation, protects against certain types of cancer and increases levels of BDNF in the brain

N-acetylcysteine - A powerful agent for increasing levels of glutathione

Milk thistle - A powerful liver herb that also increases levels of glutathione

Omega 3 (fish oil and/or krill oil) - A virtually compulsory supplement that supports brain and heart health along with reducing levels of systemic inflammation

Alpha lipoic acid - Another powerful supplement for increasing glutathione

Caloric restriction

Possibly the most potent way to slow down biological aging is unfortunately also the least palatable for most people - myself included. Studies have consistently showed that by dramatically reducing the number of calories a mouse or a human consumes, a raft of biological changes occur which leads to slow aging.

However my view would probably be shared by most people - any life where I can't eat the things I love is not worth living. I would probably last a month or so on caloric restriction before I would die tragically in a self-inflicted, shotgun-related mishap.

According to Eric Ravussin, a human health and performance researcher at the Pennington Biomedical Research Center in Louisiana, 15% less calories from age 25 could bestow upon you a grand total of 4 and a half years extra longevity. *No thanks.*

Even if you decide that you can handle the idea of lifelong caloric restriction, the majority of people soon give up, tired of feeling hungry all the time. It's no way to live.

A more palatable but less potent way of mimicking the effects of caloric restriction would be via resveratrol supplementation, which appears to work via similar mechanisms, as mentioned earlier in this book.

But perhaps a better option for those that can handle it would be to try one of the various forms of intermittent fasting, which involves periods of low or no calories interspersed with normal eating.

Intermittent fasting has compelling research results to back it up as a means to extend lifespan. It appears to -

1. Reduce oxidative damage - It is theorized that when you are fasting and your body is not dedicating its internal resources to the process of digestion, it is able to dedicate those resources to repair work.

2. Increase insulin sensitivity - This leads to less incidence of type 2 diabetes and other problems caused by high blood sugar

3. Improved mitochondrial function

In general, intermittent fasting appears to act via the same mechanism I mentioned in the section on stress - *hormesis*. It is a kind of small, survivable shock to the organism that increases its overall robustness and resistance to disease.

More specifically, the most obvious mechanism for the beneficial effects of intermittent fasting appears to be the effects on IGF-1 (*insulin-like growth factor 1*). This kind of fasting decreases the expression of IGF-1 (which is called "insulin-like" because it has a similar molecular structure to insulin), a hormone that is central to the anabolic growth of cells. Deficiencies in either IGF-1 or human growth hormone (which is largely controlled by IGF-1) result in stunted growth problems. According to Professor Valter Longo of the University of Southern California, by decreasing the expression of IGF-1, there is a temporary switch from a growth focus to a repair focus, leading to less damage accumulating over the longer term.

So how important is IGF-1 to longevity? Mice bred to have very low levels of IGF-1 expression live for 40% longer than their standard counterparts. What about humans with low levels of IGF-1 expression? That would be the people with the rare condition *Laron syndrome*, who have unusually low levels of IGF-1 expression. As you would expect, they are much smaller than the average person as they lack the growth hormone mediated anabolic effects we typically have. However, slightly more surprising is the fact that sufferers of Laron syndrome experience much lower rates of diabetes and cancer. Clearly, IGF-1 is a powerful mediator of longevity and our most powerful means to achieve reduced IGF-1 expression at the moment is intermittent fasting.

The other attractive benefit of intermittent fasting for longevity, is that it can lead to often dramatic weight loss. This flies in the face of previously accepted wisdom that recommended regular small meals as the best way to lose weight because this "stokes the fires of your metabolism". The tide of opinion is gradually turning against this line of thinking. This is due partly to the fact that most people's experience is that intermittent fasting sheds weight more effectively, but also due to what we are now learning about the longevity-enhancing effects of periods of time spent without eating food.

How you implement intermittent fasting is largely up to you, as the key appears to be the calories cut rather than any particular way in which each block of eating and fasting is constructed. You can either try - *alternate day fasting* (ADF) which involves one day of normal eating followed by a day of fasting, or the *5:2 diet*, which involves two ultra-low calorie days (they must not be on consecutive days) and five days of normal eating.

Personally I have tried the 5:2 diet and while I found it easier than I expected, it was not something I felt I could maintain for any meaningful period of time. If you want to try this, experiment with what works for you. The key is to find the option that requires the least amount of willpower, as this will be the option with the highest chances of success for you personally.

Get good quality sleep

The connection between stress, elevated cortisol levels and a host of negative health consequences is reasonably well known. What is less widely known is that regularly sleeping less than six hours per night has the exact same effects on the body as chronic stress, including increased cortisol, systemic inflammation and a weakened immune system.

The problem is that this situation applies to more than 30% of all Americans. I don't have any data on the rest of the western world, however I would hazard a guess that the rate is roughly similar when averaged out.

The biggest study into the link between sleep duration and mortality found that sleeping less than six hours per night was associated with a 12% increase in risk of death. Where it gets really interesting is when we see that sleeping more than nine hours per night is associated with a 30% increase in risk of death!

However we need to remember than correlation doesn't equal causation. For example, poor health can cause increased sleep duration in some cases, which would account for the increased risk of death. Similarly, a painful or disabling health condition could be impacting sleep, leading to less time spent asleep.

What we do know however, is that deliberately depriving an animal of sleep can lead to its swift demise. Other studies where subjects are allowed to sleep but are woken as soon as they enter deep (slow wave) sleep also show interesting results. Even though these subjects are getting some of the stages of sleep, without slow wave sleep they literally fall apart, with severe fatigue and even widespread pain that mimics fibromyalgia (*As an aside, the fact that depriving a healthy subject of slow wave sleep appears to cause temporary fibromyalgia, this points to a possible mechanism, among many others, behind this disorder*)

Conservatively however, if we accept these numbers on face value, it would be safe to assume that somewhere between six and nine hours is the "sweet spot" in terms of sleep duration and longevity.

If we look at all the negative health consequences of chronic sleep deprivation, we see an eerie correlation with stress. Sleep deprivation appears to act as a kind of stressor, leading to all the same problems. The main difference is that sleep deprivation manages to achieve all the nasty stuff that stress does, but in a fraction of the time. While the effects of chronic stress slowly build over time, just a few nights of little or no sleep can break even the most durable mind. It's no coincidence that sleep deprivation is an effective torture technique.

There is a kind of "chicken and the egg" relationship between sleep and mental illness.

Sleep deprivation is a strong trigger for mental illness and mental illness itself leads to sleep disorders (early morning awakenings, insomnia etc.). Considering that it is during slow wave sleep when your neurotransmitters and hormones (particularly growth hormone) undergo their main process of replenishment, getting insufficient sleep is a recipe for disaster.

What is less clear is the importance of REM (rapid eye movement) sleep on longevity, as the function of REM sleep is still not proven. What we do know, however, is that major depression is associated with increased levels of REM sleep and less slow wave sleep. As most SSRI antidepressants suppress REM sleep, some have hypothesized that suppressing REM sleep (if you have too much of it due to depression) is one of the keys to treating mood disorders. Interestingly, if you artificially prevent a depressed person from experiencing REM sleep by depriving them of sleep, their mood improves dramatically. Unfortunately, this effect only lasts until they next go to sleep - when they wake up again, their depression will remain. Complete sleep deprivation is not a particularly compliance-friendly treatment in any case.

Sleep deprivation not only leads to immediate health consequences, it also causes downstream problems. For example, a lack of sleep leads to disturbances in the appetite-related hormones ghrelin and leptin. This then leads to weight gain, causing a new constellation of problems.

But perhaps the most instantaneous of possible consequences is regarding accidents caused by sleep deprivation. These accidents can go from car accidents caused by fatigue, to the space shuttle *Challenger* disaster, which is believed to have been precipitated indirectly by sleep deprivation.

You need to prioritize sleep ahead of virtually all else, save for drinking water. Nothing will cause things to unravel quicker than sleep deprivation. Unfortunately, for many, sleep comes last in the queue - they will prioritize everything else (work, social engagements, television etc.) ahead of sleep and then sleep duration is just made up of whatever is left, time-wise.

However, sleep is not just a function of duration. Sleep quality must also be preserved and enhanced. If you drink a bottle of wine and fall into a coma for 8 hours, your sleep quality will look completely different to a typical sleep EEG (*electroencephalogram*). Alcohol is poison for sleep quality as it keeps you in the lighter stages of sleep all night. Just another reason why being an alcoholic is up there with cigarette smoking in terms of toxicity to the body and early mortality.

In terms of improving sleep quality, some keys are -

- Avoid alcohol and caffeinated beverages in the evening. Alcohol prevents you from entering into deep sleep and caffeine messes with adenosine levels. Adenosine levels gradually increase during the day and eventually signal your body to sleep at night. Caffeine inhibits this process, reducing sleep quality and often causing insomnia in susceptible individuals.

- Avoid eating too much at night. Sleep quality while digesting a heavy meal is poor.

- Practice relaxation techniques such as meditation or progressive muscle relaxation in the evening.

- Try a warm bath before bed. This has been shown to increase levels of slow wave sleep by accentuating the drop in body temperature that accompanies sleep. Because your body has to cool you down by a greater degree after a bath (as your core temperature is higher), you sleep more deeply. Scientists are still unsure why this actually works, but it does.

If you want further motivation, perhaps clinical trial results may help. Multiple studies have shown that insomniacs have significantly greater levels of oxidative stress than healthy controls (those without insomnia). For example, Gulec et al stated *"Our results show that the patients with primary insomnia had significantly lower GSH-Px activity and higher MDA levels compared with the controls"* and therefore *"These results may indicate the important role of sleep in attenuating oxidative stress"*. Whether you look at it from the perspective of cortisol or oxidative stress, not getting sufficient sleep clearly accelerates the aging process.

So what about sleeping tablets?

While many people tend to get a bit hysterical over sleeping tablets (primarily due to perceived addiction risk), I think you have to get pragmatic sometimes. If it's a choice between chronic insomnia and taking a pill, I will take a pill every time. But there are a few caveats and key points.

Sleeping tablets should be a measure of last resort or used for occasional insomnia - It's no use drinking beer and coffee every night or doing your work presentations on your laptop in bed and wondering why you can't sleep. Before you resort to sleeping tablets, make sure your house is in order in terms of sleep hygiene.

The main reasons why doctors exercise caution regarding sleeping tablets is that (in general - there are some exceptions I will get to in a moment) they give you poor quality sleep and they do carry some addiction risk.

If you visit your doctor complaining of insomnia, depending on the doctor and what country you are in, you will most likely be prescribed either a benzodiazepine (such as temazepam, diazepam or alprazolam) or one of the newer, related "z-drugs" such as zolpidem (*Ambien, Stillnox*), zaleplon (*Sonata*) or eszopiclone (*Lunesta*). There are a range of problems with benzodiazepines which mean that they are being prescribed less and less for sleep problems (they are however, extremely helpful for severe anxiety and panic disorders). They rob you of vital slow wave sleep, which can be deleterious over long periods of time. They also carry the risk of addiction or physical dependence if used at high doses for extended periods. While the risk of addiction to benzodiazepines is often overstated, you don't want to try your luck. Poly-drug users often mention that withdrawing from benzodiazepines like alprazolam (*Xanax*) or clonazepam (*Klonopin*) is worse than heroin. In fact, along with alcohol withdrawal, benzodiazepine withdrawal is one of the only other drugs where the withdrawal process can be life threatening if done incorrectly.

The beauty of z-drugs is that, while they also carry the risk of dependence, they don't wreck your sleep architecture to the same degree.

If you have severe, life-long insomnia however, the longevity-promoting effects of getting sleep will far outweigh any consequences of taking sleeping tablets for extended periods of time. However if you require indefinite assistance to help you sleep, it is better to look at options which are indicated for long term use and which don't ruin your sleep quality. Some potential options include -

Mirtazapine (*Remeron, Avanza, Zispin*) - This is an antidepressant that essentially functions as a super-potent sedating antihistamine with relatively weak antidepressant and anti-anxiety effects. If your sleep problems are caused by underlying issues with depression, this can be a good option. Mirtazapine actually improves sleep quality, in contrast to the benzodiazepines. The major downside is weight gain, which has its own health issues. Mirtazapine users have said that being on the drug is like having the perpetual "munchies".

Promethazine (*Phenergan*) or **diphenhydramine** (*Benadryl*) - These are two older sedating antihistamines which you can get OTC (over the counter) in most countries. Like mirtazapine and other antihistamines, usually improve sleep quality. Some people however react badly to antihistamines and feel groggy the next day. The best part about antihistamines is that they have a long history of safe use. You are unlikely to suddenly grow an extra leg after using them.

Pregabalin (*Lyrica*) or **gabapentin** (*Neurontin*) - These were developed as anticonvulsants but are now used mainly for neuropathic pain (such as fibromyalgia or post-herpetic neuralgia) and anxiety disorders. Both of these drugs improve sleep quality dramatically.

They appear to do this by reducing levels of excitatory neurotransmitters such as glutamate, noradrenaline (norepinephrine) and substance P. People tend to either love them or hate them, with many stopping treatment soon after beginning due to intolerable side-effects. Like mirtazapine, the other main problem is weight gain.

There are some other options as well, however for one reason or another, they are not viable. There are the older tricyclic antidepressants (such as amitriptyline), which improve sleep quality at the expense of cardiac function and anticholinergic problems. There is also sodium oxybate (*Xyrem*), which is one of the most potent drugs available for increasing slow wave sleep. The main problem is that sodium oxybate is another name for *GHB*, an illegal street drug. If you are able to successfully convince your doctor to prescribe Xyrem for you, send me their details and I will go and get some from them myself!

Remember though, that there is no such thing as a free lunch. Any extended pharmaceutical use will have consequences, no matter how benign. You just need to weigh up the consequences of this versus long term insomnia, which has deleterious effects on the brain that far outweighs even the most toxic of sleeping tablets (unless perhaps if you need to start sniffing glue to get some shut-eye).

However you need to realize that insomnia rarely occurs in a vacuum. It is generally a symptom of something else, either behavioral (you read work emails in bed just before you are about to go to sleep or something similarly non-conducive to sleep) or neurochemical (underlying depression or anxiety). Occasionally someone has some innate biological problem getting to sleep, however I believe that these people are exceedingly rare. So the best course of action generally is to address whatever is causing your insomnia, use sleeping tablets as a short term solution to get you through, and if nothing works, investigate longer-term options for pharmacological assistance.

Maintain a healthy immune system

We only have to look at HIV AIDS to see what happens when your immune system becomes compromised. However, did you know that the immune system is also responsible for controlling many types of cancer? When a cell "goes rogue" and switches off its own apoptosis (programmed cell death), it is the immune system that identifies and neutralizes the threat before it can develop into cancer.

Imagine your immune system is like a group of soldiers defending a city (your body). Whenever they find an external invader (like a bacteria or virus), they are easily identified and taken care of. However cancer cells are a little trickier. Cancer cells are like a rogue traitorous soldier who has decided to join the enemy. Because they are wearing the uniform of the "home team", they are not as easy to identify. Therefore, occasionally something slips through the defenses and can turn into a cancer.

However a key determinant of how good your immune system "soldiers" are at keeping the cancer cells at bay is overall immune function. If you have compromised immune function or a lifestyle that triggers too many cells to "go rogue", you are increasing your chances of developing cancer.

And immune function is not just related to cancer. A compromised immune system is one of the major problems associated with old age. Young, healthy subjects with full-strength immune systems don't develop pneumonia regularly. A weakened immune system is one of the fundamental hallmarks of the aging process. One of the main reasons for this is the gradual decline in your body's ability to manufacture new *T lymphocytes* (T-cells) and B *lymphocytes* (B-cells) which make up part of your front line defense.

Therefore, quite a bit of research has been directed at either reversing the atrophy of your thymus (the organ that produces T-cells – hence the "T") or reactivating white blood cells. Until recently, it was thought that white blood cells became inactive due to telomere shortening. However recent research has indicated that may not be the case and that it may be possible to re-activate the white blood cells. One of the researchers in this particular study likened it to bring football players out of retirement and back into the game.

While specific therapies emerging out of this research are some time off, we are fortunate in the meantime that we already have a variety of ways to support and regenerate immune system function. For example, if we stay on the subject of the thymus, dietary zinc supplements have been showed to have a beneficial effect on thymus size and function. A 2009 study by Wong et al found *"...that in mice, zinc supplementation can reverse some age-related thymic defects and may be of considerable benefit in improving immune function and overall health in elderly populations".*

In terms of supplementation, the following all have good, solid research backing –

Curcumin – Yes, curcumin again. Is there anything it can't do?

Garlic – There is some evidence that garlic possesses some immune-boosting effects. Due to the sulfur content, you should already be eating a diet rich in garlic anyway

Astragalus – This has a long history of use in Chinese medicine as an immune system herb. Some interesting preliminary research suggests that astragalus may increase telomerase activity. A proprietary extract of astragalus appears to reduce the extent to which T-cells become senescent and inactive.

Olive leaf extract – As well as acting as an anti-microbial (it fights bacteria, viruses and fungi), olive leaf extract also appears to stimulate phagocytosis, which is where your *macrophagocytes* (another one of your immune system's army of soldiers) attack and engulf a pathogen.

This is just a few of the various supplements and herbs which may have immune-boosting effects. There are a range of other options also, including – Echinacea, goldenseal and vitamin C.

Unfortunately however, there are no supplements that could be considered to have proven and reproducible effects on the immune system. For example, some studies have shown echinacea to be of benefit, whereas others did not.

Fortunately however, we have a much more powerful way of modulating the immune system to prevent age-related decline. Unfortunately, however, I am going to sound like a broken record because the most powerful way to maintain a healthy, functioning immune system is to manage and avoid chronic stress.

Ever noticed how, during a period of intense stress you suddenly come down with a cold? It's no co-incidence. Scientists have known for a long time now that there is a strong connection between stress levels and your immune system. Your immune system and your sympathetic nervous system (your fight or flight system that prepares you for action) have a rich network of various type of connections. For example, many of the cells that your immune system uses to fight pathogens, such as lymphocytes, have special receptors for various substances produced during periods of stress, such as noradrenaline and endorphins. Research has consistently found that stress reduces the activity of natural killer cells and suppresses the proliferation of lymphocytes.

Also, consistent with what I mentioned in the section on stress, it appears clear that time-limited, acute stress (such as the stress before an exam) enhances immune response, while chronic stress (such as an abusive relationship or a stressful job) suppresses immune response.

If you can prevent or eliminate chronic stress, you are able to ameliorate much of the age-related decline in immune response. This by no means confers a 100 year old the immune system of a teenager. There are still age-related declines in immune function that will occur in everybody. However, I am hopeful that one of the current research projects throws up a novel agent that is able to identify and mitigate the worst of our age-related decline in immune function.

Another factor which many believe to be central to immune system status is vitamin D levels. Yes, vitamin D. Again. There is a strong correlation between vitamin D levels and immune function. Some scientists believe this may be one of the factors as to why we get colds and flu more often in the winter time when we naturally get less sun exposure. So ensure that you get at least 20 minutes per day of sun exposure and take vitamin D supplements (with vitamin K as well).

Keep your brain young with *nootropics*

"Nootropics" are essentially supplements and drugs which enhance brain function in some way. In general, all nootropics work by either increasing the supply of oxygen to the brain, the production or supply of the neurotransmitters or by stimulating *neuroplastic* brain growth. The father of nootropics, Dr. Corneliu E. Giurgea, said that, by definition, nootropics –

1. Should enhance learning and memory
2. Should protect the brain from injury or damage
3. Should improve brain functioning
4. Should be relatively safe for the brain and be without serious side-effects

In terms of drugs, currently the most widely used nootropics are the various stimulants used to treat ADHD including *methylphenidate* and *amphetamine*. These drugs enhance cognitive function by improving concentration, reducing impulsive behavior and improving planning skills. However in my opinion (except in rare circumstances) I think that ADHD-related stimulants fail point 4) above as I don't believe they are a completely safe long term option for improving cognition or memory for most people.

Often, the difference between stimulants and other drugs used to treat diseases such as Parkinson's and Huntington's is vague. In general, all of these drugs work by different means to modulate levels of either dopamine or norepinephrine.

Different nootropics work via different means. For example, gingko appears to work by increasing blood flow to the brain, with all the benefits that increased blood supply brings. However, most nootropics work to improve mental function by modulating key neurotransmitters including acetylcholine, dopamine, norepinephrine and glutamate. Of these, acetylcholine and dopamine are central to most processes that improve cognitive function.

Acetylcholine is your most abundant neurotransmitter, due mainly to the face that it is located not only in the central nervous system (your brain, essentially) by also can be found in the peripheral nervous system (the rest of your body). In the body, acetylcholine is required for muscle activation, including your vital breathing function. To demonstrate how important this neurotransmitter is, certain lethal nerve gases such as *sarin* (used recently in Syria on innocent women and children) work by impairing the action of acetylcholine. In the brain, acetylcholine works to modulate attention and arousal (meaning physiological, not sexual in this context).

Dopamine, along with norepinephrine and glutamate, is one of the brain's key excitatory neurotransmitters. Dopamine is an interesting substance; being involved centrally in staying focused and motivated, along with being vital to the process of moving your body. The movement disorder Parkinson's, involves the death of dopamine producing neurons in the part of the brain responsible for movement. Put another way, evolution has made it so that dopamine moves you (both physically and mentally) towards goals that are beneficial for your survival.

The way that dopamine achieves this is by giving you a sensation of pleasure in anticipating something rewarding. That little burst of pleasure you feel in anticipation of a delicious meal or 'sexy time' with a potential partner is due to dopamine.

As dopamine helps you focus on your goals, low levels of dopamine can lead to conditions such as ADD and ADHD, where a lack of dopamine (and norepinephrine) leads to an inability to concentrate on certain tasks. Drugs like methylphenidate help alleviate the symptoms of ADD by increasing levels of dopamine (and again norepinephrine to a lesser extent).

The granddaddy of all nootropics is a class of supplements called *racetams*. This is surprising in as much as the majority of people have never even heard of either racetams or the most popular single example - *piracetam*.

All racetams including piracetam, pramiracetam, aniracetam as well as oxiracetam have a 2-pyrrolidone nucleus comprised of oxygen, nitrogen and hydrogen. Whilst this is the subject of a little controversy, the general consensus is that racetams work by stimulating production of acetylcholine and/or by improving the uptake of glutamate by activating AMPA and NDMA receptors. As acetylcholine and glutamate are central to enhancing neural function, it is not surprising then that racetams can have dramatic effects in terms of improved cognitive function.

Piracetam

Interestingly, piracetam is a distant relative of GABA (the neurotransmitter affected by drugs such as benzodiazepines to reduce anxiety) and was originally developed with the intention that it would be a potential treatment for anxiety. However early studies showed that rather than acting as an anxiolytic (anxiety reducing), it appeared to improve cognitive function and protect the brain against certain damage such as that caused by dementia or lack of oxygen. It was soon apparent that the mechanism of action was closely linked to glutamate activity at the NMDA and AMPA receptors along with modulation of the cholinergic system.

The NMDA receptor is central to your brain's process of learning and adaptation via neural plasticity. If we cast our minds back, we may remember that up until recently, scientists believed that the brain was fixed at birth and could not be altered in structure. However all that changed with the discovery of *neurogenesis* (the birth of new brain cells) and *neuroplasticity*. Now we know that you can change your brain by repetitive behaviors (a concept harnessed by *cognitive behavioral therapy*) and by selective modulation of particular brain systems, of which the NMDA receptor is central.

Activating the NMDA receptor also stimulates increased levels of *brain derived neurotrophic factor* (BDNF), which, as I mentioned before, has been described as a kind of fertilizer for the brain. The stimulation of BDNF is thought to be one of the reasons why cardiovascular exercise and antidepressant drugs alleviate depression. As a central theme in your own research, anything which is positive for BDNF is usually positive for your brain.

The other means by which we can see how important the NMDA receptor is for learning is when we decrease its activity via drugs known as NMDA receptor antagonists, which includes street drugs PCP and the popular cough-suppressant dextromethorphan (*Robitussin*). NMDA receptor antagonists have a clear effect of reducing memory formation, further reinforcing the evidence showing how vital this particular receptor is for learning.

As well as the above effects on the brain's glutaminergic system, piracetam also has beneficial effects on the cholinergic system by increasing levels of acetylcholine. Acetylcholine is also vital for cognitive function and memory storage. One of the downsides of the older style antidepressants (such as tricyclic antidepressants) was the negative effects on the cholinergic system, which impaired cognition and memory for many people taking these drugs. Likewise, we also clearly understand the important role that acetylcholine plays in this area due to the fact that diseases such as Alzheimer's appear to be caused primarily by problems with receptor density (the number of these receptors decreases) along with a decrease in acetylcholine levels in particular parts of the brain. Indeed, newer drugs for Alzheimer's patients focus on addressing this issue in the cholinergic system to restore mental functioning.

Recent research has shown the action of piracetam may be linked to another factor unrelated to acetylcholine. This research has indicated that piracetam may exert its beneficial effects on the brain via its ability to improve the structure of the brain's cell membranes. Piracetam appears to improve the fluidity and permeability (the ability for certain substances to go in and out of the cell), thus improving certain cognitive functions which rely on this smooth transfer between the inside and outside of your brain's cells.

One of my favorite stacks cantered on piracetam is to add co-enzyme Q10 (CoQ10). Many of the nasty side-effects associated with anti-cholesterol drugs (statins) such as Lipitor and Crestor are linked to a depletion of CoQ10. CoQ10 is a vital co-factor for healthy mitochondria, which are your body's cellular powerhouses (and central to some of the main theories on why we age). CoQ10, when paired with piracetam, which improves the structure of the mitochondrial cell walls, provide a potent nootropic powerhouse in my experience.

As previously mentioned, one of the ways by which piracetam appears to work is by enhancing the brain's cholinergic system. This is done by both increasing the density of acetylcholine receptors in the brain and by increasing circulating levels of acetylcholine. One of my favorite nootropics, acetyl-L-carnitine (ALCAR) also works partially by increasing levels of glutamate receptors in the brain. ALCAR appears to work together with piracetam to increase levels of acetylcholine by increasing levels of an important enzyme called *choline acetyl transferase.*

Another angle to consider is to increase levels of choline in the brain via consumption of certain foods or supplements. You can consume a large amount of foods such as eggs or take choline supplements. However my preference is to take CDP choline (or citicoline) or alpha GPC - both of which have been proven to increase levels of choline in the brain more potently than pure choline supplementation alone.

Like many aspects of nootropics, I believe these effects are most pronounced in those over

50 years of age who may have already begun a certain degree of cognitive decline. Piracetam in combination with ALCAR and CoQ10 appears to be a potent ally in the fight against the common cognitive aspects of aging.

Users report clear improvements in various aspects of brain functioning including attention and motivation – effects clearly consistent with its relationship to the brain's acetylcholine system.

In terms of dosage, most use between 1-3 grams per day, however you may need to experiment with dosage to find your own sweet spot.

Acetyl L-Carnitine (ALCAR)

As I mentioned previously, ALCAR is a potent supplement for improving mental function - particularly in combination with a racetam. The primary mechanism of action appears to be by optimizing levels of acetylcholine, however it also appears to improve mood and motivation via its positive effects on the brain's dopamine system. It is for this reason that ALCAR has been studied as a potential supplement for reducing some of the debilitating effects of Parkinson's disease. Early studies have been quite promising.

ALCAR also acts as a powerful antioxidant in the brain, repairing damage caused by lifestyle and natural aging. This is likely to be one of the reasons why it has shown great potential as a treatment for fibromyalgia, a condition associated with accelerated brain aging due to chronic stress (this is the same reason why the anti-dementia drug *memantine* has been studied as a treatment for fibromyalgia - due to its ability repair damage caused by stress and an overactive glutaminergic system).

ALCAR also demonstrates a great synergistic effect when taken with CoQ10, increasing energy levels via positive effects on your mitochondria. It also appears to enhance neuroplastic healing, as there have been studies showing a beneficial effect for the recovery from strokes, where ALCAR appeared to accelerate brain healing.

Phosphatidylserine (PS)

As we discussed in the section on racetams, the membrane of your cell walls is vitally important for enhanced cognitive function. A healthy cell wall enables smooth and efficient transfer of information between the inside and outside of each cell. One of the major components of the cell wall is a substance called phosphatidylserine (PS).

Supplementation with PS appears to be particularly beneficial for conditions involving poor concentration and memory, such as ADHD. PS also showed promise in a study looking at its possible use as a treatment for depression. My suspicion is that PS would only be useful to treat depression for a particular sub-set of the disorder. Remember - depression is not a single illness but a collection of symptoms. Based on the way that PS works, I think it would be useful for depression related to cell wall dysfunction or lack of permeability, along with depression caused by chronically elevated cortisol. As you may know, cortisol is a major hormone associated with the stress response. After a period of protracted, chronic stress, levels of cortisol can be consistently high with depression often resulting, depending on the individual's particular genetic makeup.

N-Acetylcysteine (NAC)

I have already talked about NAC extensively in terms of the benefits to the liver and as a way to increase levels of glutathione. However, just like alpha lipoic acid, NAC is incredibly beneficial for the brain as a general damage repairer and detoxifier.

In terms of specific disorders, NAC has shown great promise for treating obsessive compulsive disorder (OCD) by decreasing levels of certain neurotransmitters which keep the sufferer's brain locked at 'full speed'. Incredibly, NAC is also garnering interest from scientists as a potential treatment for schizophrenia and bipolar disorder.

Due to the fact that NAC can have quite powerful effects on the brain, you should exercise caution. Anecdotally, I have heard many stories from users who either said it made them feel fantastic or feel worse than they did before. It all comes down to your particular brain state and how NAC works with it. If you start to take NAC and notice you feel worse, discontinue and focus your efforts elsewhere.

Choline, alpha GPC & citicoline (CDP choline)

As I mentioned in the section on racetams, I prefer alpha GPC and citicoline over straight choline as a means to provide nootropic effects. Both alpha GPC and citicoline are closely related to choline, however with a slightly different structure which enables them to cross the blood brain barrier and exert positive effects on the brain.

This group of supplements is vital to a myriad of different processes in the brain, from the production of acetylcholine to the repair of the cell membrane itself. However each has a slightly different profile.

One of the main unique benefits of citicoline is its ability to increase the density of dopamine receptors in the brain. As previously mentioned, dopamine is central to motivation and focus and dysfunction is implicated in conditions such as ADHD. Studies have shown significant improvements in memory formation and recall for subjects taking citicoline. And perhaps even more promisingly, citicoline has demonstrated the ability to reverse some of the brain damage associated with Alzheimer's disease.

The dopaminergic effects of citicoline also mean it has been used successfully to reduce drug cravings for recovering cocaine addicts. Chronic consumption of large amounts of cocaine can lead to significant dysfunction of the dopamine system, so this is quite promising and provides further evidence for citicoline's beneficial effects on the brain.

Alpha GPC has also shown plenty of promise in trials. Like its relative citicoline, alpha GPC has demonstrated a potent ability to improve memory and cognitive function not only in healthy individuals but also in Alzheimer's sufferers.

All three of these choline-related substances also have beneficial effects on mood due to the fact that they are used by the body to synthesize *trimethylglycine* (TMG) and *s-adenosylmethionine* (SAM-e), two substances which are central to maintaining healthy levels of key neurotransmitters such as serotonin, dopamine and norepinephrine. You may have heard of SAM-e due to its use as a natural antidepressant. Unsurprisingly, a study showed a strong link between low levels of choline in the diet and levels of anxiety.

The major dietary source of choline is eggs, which I believe to be one of nature's true 'super foods'. Eggs are a nutritional powerhouse and should form a key component of any non-vegan's diet. Unfortunately, whilst eggs are a great way to maintain healthy levels of choline in your diet, they do not contain enough to be used therapeutically and therefore supplementation may be required. But keep eating those eggs anyway!

This is particularly the case if you are an expectant mother or planning on conceiving soon. A recent study showed a strong correlation between a mother's consumption of choline and the IQ of her child. Now, with many study, we don't know for sure which direction the arrow of causation travels. Does choline directly increase the IQ of children because their mother consumes enough of it, or do intelligent women tend to have more nutritious and healthy diets high in choline?

Choline has also shown the ability to reduce brain damage associated with severe alcoholism. Indeed, many swear that the best possible hangover cure is a big serving of eggs, which are jam packed with choline.

If that wasn't enough, like several of the other nootropics I mention, the above three choline-related supplements increase levels of glutathione and reduce inflammation, thereby provide generalized assistance to healing a damaged and inflamed brain.

Inositol

Inositol is a type of sugar which is often bunched together with B-Group vitamins or choline, despite the fact that it is unrelated to either. Inositol has gained some attention recently when a trial using high doses showed strong benefit as an antidepressant agent and also as a potential treatment for OCD, bipolar and panic disorder.

Inositol appears to work by enhancing smooth neurotransmission, allowing better flow of the key neurotransmitters involved in mood disorders.

Inositol and choline are often sold together as a single supplement due to the fact that they appear to work synergistically, each increasing the effects of the other.

Huperzine-A

Another supplement which falls in the category of those that few have heard of is huperzine-A.

Huperzine-A has been gaining positive attention from researchers recently as a potential treatment for Alzheimer's due to the fact that, like the drug memantine, it reduces damage caused by too much glutamate activity. Huperzine-A, again similar to memantine, functions as an NMDA receptor antagonist and also increases levels of acetylcholine in the brain. Further increasing its credibility as a powerful nootropic, Huperzine A also increases levels of nerve growth factor

B-Group Vitamins

This is probably the most boring supplement listed here but one I can't omit. So many of your brain's various functions and reactions requires one of the B-group vitamins that if you are deficient in any of them, optimal neural functioning will be impossible.

As you may know, B vitamins are not a single vitamin but a whole group of vitamins which are grouped together as a class with the major link being the fact that they are water-soluble. Vitamins are usually either fat soluble (vitamin D, vitamin A, vitamin E etc.) or water soluble (vitamin C and B group vitamins) with some rare exceptions such as alpha lipoic acid which is both. The reason why it is important to know that B vitamins are water soluble is the fact that this means your body cannot store them and needs to constantly replenish levels through your diet. This is what makes B group vitamins an important supplement as it is difficult to ensure you get the right amount each and every day. Vitamin D is stored in the body so if you go without sunshine for a few days it is no big deal. However if you were to consume no B group vitamins for a few days, you would definitely notice significant mental and cognitive impairment.

Any supplement you can buy which has a mix of different vitamins and other substances to fight stress will always have B group vitamins. This is not only because B vitamins are used to synthesize stress-fighting neurotransmitters, but chronic stress has been shown to deplete levels of certain B group vitamins also. Alcoholism also drains the B-group vitamins. Indeed, you are recommended to take a nice large Mega B when you get home from a big night of drinking. It really should go without saying however I will anyway - alcohol is absolutely horrendous for the brain and if you are reading this book while remaining either an alcoholic or a binge drinker, you are wasting your time. Alcohol and longevity don't mix.

Unless you have a specific condition which requires large amounts of a single B group vitamins, I just recommend you take a single 'multi-B' each day to cover off on your requirements.

Here are the main B-group vitamins -

Thiamine (B1)
Thiamine is vital for healthy brain metabolism and for the production of acetylcholine. As a guide on how important thiamine is for a healthy brain, you only have to look at what happens when the brain is chronically deficient in thiamine - debilitating diseases such as beriberi and *Wernicke-Korsakoff syndrome*.

Riboflavin (B2)
Riboflavin is vital for synthesizing our old buddy glutathione and should therefore be a priority to ensure you have sufficient amounts in your diet or via supplementation.

Niacin (B3)
A recent study showed that niacin offers a degree of protection against Alzheimer's and other types of age-related cognitive decline syndromes. It has also been used to accelerate the brain's healing after certain types of strokes.

Just like with thiamine, as a guide to what can happen if you are chronically deficient in niacin, just look up the dreaded disease called Pellagra which was caused by diets deficient in niacin.

Pantothenic Acid (B5)

Pantothenic acid is one of the co-factors involved in acetylcholine production and unsurprisingly, research has shown that supplementation can provide tangible benefits for memory recall and concentration.

Pyridoxine (B6)

Pyridoxine is essential for the production of neurotransmitters such as serotonin, dopamine and noradrenaline. Therefore it comes as no surprise that deficiency of Pyridoxine has been strongly implicated in mood disorders such as depression and anxiety.

Biotin (B7)

Biotin, one of the lesser-known B-group vitamins, is vital for the metabolism of fatty acids in the brain - a process central to optimal brain functioning. Indeed brain cells at an individual level require sufficient levels of biotin, with deficiency potentially leading to seizures. That said, I believe actual biotin deficiency to be exceedingly rare and you would generally obtain enough from your diet.

Folic Acid (B9)

Folic Acid (or folate) is perhaps the most well-known of the B-group vitamins due to the fact that expecting mothers are recommended to take folic acid supplements to prevent neural tube defects in their baby. Folic acid is also vital for the production of serotonin. In fact, a form of folic acid is sometimes prescribed as an adjunct to antidepressant drugs to increase their effectiveness. The reasoning is that folic acid helps more serotonin go into the 'serotonin tank' and antidepressant drugs (typically SSRI class drugs such as fluoxetine, sertraline or escitalopram) act to prevent leakage from the tank (yes, this is gross oversimplification but will suffice as a rough analogy).

One thing to bear in mind is that a certain subset of the population are unable to metabolize folic acid correctly and will require it in the form of L-methylfolate. If you are suffering from a mood disorder or have been taking an SSRI with little effect, it may be worth trying a trial of L-methylfolate. If you then feel your mood lifting, it will tell you that you are part of the subset of the population with this folate conversion issue.

Cobalamin (B12)

Whist there are no studies which have been conducted using cobalamin to treat a particular illness, there have been some interesting studies showing associations. Among these was a study showing that a B12 deficiency leads to poor results on cognitive tests and another study showing a linkage between high consumption of B12 and lower incidence of Alzheimer's disease. B12 deficiency, which is extremely common in the vegetarian and vegan population, has also been strongly linked to symptoms of lethargy, poor sleep and general motivational issues.

B12 is poorly absorbed from typical food sources such as red meat, so if you are diagnosed as deficient in B12, you will need to have a course of B12 injections or at the very least, take a separate sublingual B12 (by dissolving the tablet under your tongue, you bypass your usual metabolism which leads to little being absorbed). All vegetarians and vegans should get themselves tested for B12 deficiency, however for typical meat eaters consuming a balanced diet, a clinically diagnosed deficiency is rare.

Mucuna Pruriens, L-Phenylalanine & L-Tyrosine

As I have mentioned previously, the neurotransmitter dopamine is vital for certain higher cognitive functions such as focus and abstract thought. However more is not always better, as Parkinson's patients would well know. Too little dopamine and you experience depression, lack of motivation, lack of focus and inability to feel pleasure. Too much dopamine and you can start hallucinating. Remember, many of the anti-psychotic drugs used to treat schizophrenia work by reducing levels of dopamine.

However I am really only talking about extremes here. In general, my experience has been that giving your dopamine levels a little boost is usually a powerful way to upgrade your cognitive abilities. Naturally, the various drugs that modulate dopamine are the most powerful way to achieve this, however they come with side-effects. Fortunately there are also supplemental options. Which route you go down will depend on your particular situation. If a lack of dopamine production is behind your lack of focus or motivation, then several amino acids and a powerful Indian herb may help.

L-phenylalanine and L-tyrosine are the amino acid building blocks of dopamine. They are relatively cheap and with few side-effects so definitely worth a shot as your first port of call if you suspect you are low in dopamine. However, one thing to bear in mind is that if you suffer from anxiety, I strongly caution you against using these (or any other dopamine-boosting drug or supplement for that matter). Your brain has a finely tuned balance between dopamine (and its close relative norepinephrine) and serotonin. Serotonin is made from another amino acid called L-tryptophan (or, if you go one step further in the process, 5-htp). Tryptophan is much scarcer and competes with tyrosine and phenylalanine to cross into the brain so if you supplement with these amino acids while already anxious (a state highly correlated with low serotonin), this can exacerbate the situation.

The step between tyrosine/phenylalanine and dopamine has a step in between called L-DOPA, which is the substance given to Parkinson's patients to alleviate symptoms. Interestingly, a traditional Indian herb called *mucuna pruriens* is high in L-DOPA and has also been used with some success to treat Parkinsonian symptoms. Many people swear by the cognitive enhancing effects of mucuna pruriens. I tried it for a while but did not see any dramatic results however I tend to be a naturally high dopamine person (and slightly low serotonin as a baseline). The other key point worth pointing out is that anything which increases dopamine also tends to increase libido and Mucuna Pruriens has long been used in India as an aphrodisiac. As if you didn't need any more convincing...!

Theanine

Theanine is the amino acid found primarily in tea which is reportedly responsible for the feeling of relaxed alertness associated with consuming this beverage. Theanine has some fantastic research behind it, showing that it increases dopamine, improves cognition, reduces feelings of stress and promotes alpha-waves in the brain. Also, like memantine and other similar drugs which are effective for Alzheimer's, theanine also appears to reduce damage caused by an overactive glutaminergic system.

Curcumin

Apart from acting as a general anti-inflammatory and anti-cancer agent, curcumin also possesses some fantastic properties for enhancing cognitive function and brain health. Curcumin does so many beneficial things in so many different parts of the body, my friends are all sick of me talking about it!

A recent study showed clear benefit for treating Alzheimer's patients with curcumin. As well as reducing inflammation, curcumin appears to modulate the beta-amyloid plaque responsible for this disease.

It is the anti-inflammatory aspect which is also behind curcumin's recent rise as a potential future depression treatment. The other day I was listening to the radio in my car when there was an interview with a scientist from a local prestigious hospital here in my hometown. He was invited on the show because they were conducting a study into a new hope for treating depression. Surprise, surprise – turns out it was curcumin! The scientist indicated that they had already seen positive results.

How does curcumin treat depression? This is where it gets interesting as it attacks depression from several different angles. Firstly, it reduces inflammation. Increasingly, many researchers are starting to believe that inflammation and depression are closely linked. It has long been known that depressed people have higher levels of certain pro-inflammatory biomarkers. We still don't know whether it is causation or correlation however there is a definite link. Curcumin, by reducing inflammation, appears to act as a potent antidepressant.

Secondly, curcumin functions as a MAOI, which, as previously mentioned, inhibits the action of an enzyme which breaks down serotonin, norepinephrine and dopamine in your brain, thereby increasing levels. Traditional pharmaceutical MAOIs were extremely dangerous in overdose or if you consumed certain foods like aged cheese or red wine which could trigger a hypertensive crisis. Fortunately, curcumin is known as a *reversible MAOI* so doesn't have the same health risks.

Curcumin also increases levels of BDNF, that wonderful *brain fertilizer* I mentioned before. You may have heard that cardio exercise has been found to be an excellent treatment for depression. One of the reasons for this is thought to be that exercise is a potent stimulator of BDNF levels. In depressed patients, often a smaller hippocampus is seen. The hippocampus, as well as being strongly related to memory and context detection, is strongly implicated in depression also. It is thought that by increasing levels of BDNF, you are helping your brain to 'regrow' after a bout of depression.

Sensible use of medication where appropriate

There is an old saying that says the only difference between a poison and a medicine is the dose. 1 tablet (500mg) of acetaminophen (paracetamol) will relieve pain and reduce a fever. Take twenty of them and you risk liver failure and death.

People can sometimes become too fundamental and dogmatic regarding pharmaceuticals. Yes, pharmaceuticals are largely developed by "Big Pharma" with profit in mind, but the end result is that they often reduce suffering in the world.

There is no *one size fits all* blanket statement that one can make regarding pharmaceuticals. The key question you need to ask yourself is - *Am I reducing my life expectancy by taking this drug or not taking this drug?* Sure, many drugs can have negative effects on the body (particularly the liver and brain), but these effects need to be weighed up against the alternative.

Here are some general guidelines for certain types of medications -

Statins

Statins are not inherently "evil" as some people make them out to be. They have just been misused by the marketing department of pharmaceutical companies. If you have already had a heart attack, been diagnosed with a form of heart disease or suffer from hypercholesterolemia (unhealthily high natural cholesterol levels), statins have been proven to save lives. The problem comes with the marketing. Pharmaceutical companies cleverly realized that if they could get the definition of "high cholesterol" and "at risk person" widened, they could dramatically increase the market size for statins. What has happened since has been one of the most deviously brilliant marketing and lobbying campaigns in the history of medicine. So now we have a situation where someone can visit the doctor with slightly elevated cholesterol and be put on statins. Statins have demonstrated no statistically significant ability to reduce the risk of heart disease in healthy people. However, if you are one of the at risk groups mentioned above, statins can be a lifesaver and a compulsory medicine. Don't form a dogmatic view against statins that prevents you from getting adequate care. Take time to educate yourself on the risk/benefit ratio. You need to weigh up the potential benefit of preventing a heart attack with the increased risk of diabetes, dementia or muscle problems that some researchers have linked to statins. As an interesting aside, researchers are now saying that the reason why statins can be beneficial for some is that they act as anti-inflammatories. If this is the case, personally, I would stick to omega 3, vitamin D and curcumin supplements to achieve the same result but without the side-effects.

If you do decide to take statins, please ensure you also take CoQ10 at the same time and get adequate vitamin D from the sun and also vitamin D supplements.

SSRI antidepressants

Another area where people can get infuriatingly dogmatic. At one end of the spectrum you have people who believe that antidepressants are evil and cause brain damage. At the other end you have those who believe that depression can be explained simply in terms of monoamine neurotransmitters such as serotonin. As with anything, the truth lies somewhere in the middle.

So, let me cut through the spin to lay down some simple facts -

Antidepressants work for most people to treat symptoms of depression and/or anxiety. If in doubt, don't generate your opinion based on what you read on internet forums. Internet forums on depression feature something called selection bias, which means they are not an accurate reflection of reality. The people who are on depression forums complaining that their antidepressants don't work give a skewed picture of reality. This is because if you take antidepressants and get better, you won't spend your time on the internet talking about your experience. You will have moved on.

Antidepressants don't cause brain damage - If anything, they have been proven to do the opposite. SSRI (selective serotonin reuptake inhibitors such as *Prozac, Zoloft* and *Lexapro*) therapy is associate with areas of the brain (primarily the hippocampus) re-growing, after depression has initially caused atrophy. SSRIs increased levels of BDNF, your brain's important "fertilizer".

Antidepressants don't "cure" depression. Firstly, there is no such thing as *curing* depression, only achieving *remission*. Secondly, treating depression should be done holistically, looking at - cognition, behavior, diet and other factors. Sitting back and waiting for a pill to do all the hard work is not only less effective, but means that when you go off your drugs, you are more likely to become depressed again. Depression is (in most cases) caused by something. You have to fix whatever that *something* is. A pill doesn't do that.

Depression is not "caused" by low serotonin - Depression is a hugely complex beast that still eludes a clean and simple explanation. So many different biological and psychological systems are involved that, to reduce everything down to serotonin is misguided. We don't even clearly know whether low serotonin causes depression or depression causes low serotonin. Likewise, while we know that SSRIs work, many scientists believe they work for reasons completely independent of serotonin. For example, there is a drug called tianeptine *(Stablon)*, which acts as a selective serotonin reuptake enhancer and works as an effective antidepressant. That's right - it does the exact opposite thing in your brain to SSRIs (which inhibit the reuptake of serotonin), yet treats depression. The brain is infinitely more complex than we can imagine.

Depression can be deadly. Depending on the figures you use, there are between 30,000 and 50,000 suicide deaths each year in the US alone. To withhold appropriate treatment because of dogmatic opposition or worries about the health consequences of SSRIs is insane. SSRIs have no proven link with lowered life expectancy apart from the small number of people who commit suicide shortly after beginning treatment.

However, I should also point out, that for mild to moderate cases of depression, drugs don't perform any better than placebo. Interestingly, the most effective treatment for mild to moderate depression is also one of the potent anti-agers mentioned earlier - cardiovascular exercise. In Jump Start - An introduction to the science of exercise therapy for anxiety & depression, Benjamin Kramer says *"Study after study has clearly shown that cardiovascular exercise and/or weight training works just as well as antidepressant medication, but with one key advantage - Those subjects who treat their anxiety and depression with exercise tend to stay well, whereas those who treat their depression with medication have a significantly higher relapse rate".*

Prescription stimulants for ADHD

If there was ever a candidate for the most controversial area of modern psychopharmacology, it would be the use of stimulants (such as methylphenidate and amphetamine-related drugs) to treat ADD and ADHD.

Firstly, yes, these stimulants are, in some ways, toxic for the brain. You would never take these drugs to achieve lasting, positive change in the brain.

Secondly, yes, they probably are over-prescribed - used in milder cases where behavioral intervention would be more appropriate.

However, if you have ever had any experience with the use of these drugs to treat more severe cases of ADHD, you would know that they are usually spectacularly successful. They can (in less than an hour) cause the most dramatic improvements in functioning imaginable. They can take a child, who is being both self-destructive and destructive to those around them, and create a normal, placid, fully-functioning child. The changes that can occur are sometimes nothing short of amazing. Families who have gotten their life back thanks to these medications understandably get angry when they read an academic or journalist claim that these drugs aren't helpful or that ADHD doesn't even exist.

Some believe that ADHD itself is an invented illness. Sure, this may be the case. However in my opinion, more weight must be given to the reduction in suffering of these kids than to any problems with the theory behind ADHD.

If you or your children are unable to function or lead a normal life due to the range of symptoms we call "ADHD" or "ADD", the negative effects on longevity of taking these drugs would be far outweighed by the longevity-shortening effects of not seeking appropriate pharmacological help.

Vaccines

To be honest, I find it amazing that I even have to mention vaccines. There is a special place in hell reserved for parents who refuse to vaccinate their child. The most frustrating part is that the only reason there are people suspicious of vaccines is because of a study in the UK that was later proven to be fraudulent. This fraudulent research paper garnered significant media attention and led to an immediate drop in vaccinations by panicked parents because it appeared to show that vaccines cause autism. This was predictably followed by an increase in the number of reported cases of measles and mumps.

However, here is where things get truly bizarre. Despite the fact that this study was universally proven to be fraudulent (by all but the most whacko of conspiracy theorists), the idea that vaccines cause autism remained in the minds of certain parents. This is the equivalent of someone telling you there is a bogeyman in your closet, then admitting they were only joking, yet you continue to believe the bogeyman is there.

Get your child vaccinated. End of story. According to the World Health Organisation (WHO), 2.5 million deaths are prevented each year by vaccines.

However, there are countless other medications and conditions that may need medicating - this is just a few of the main ones. Remember, everyone is different. For someone with ADHD, taking a stimulant medication can be longevity enhancing (because benefits across multiple parts of their life can outweigh the negative consequences of stimulants). For someone without ADHD, these drugs are just toxic stimulants.

If you have a health condition, get appropriate treatment (whether with drugs or otherwise). If not, stay away from unnecessary pharmaceuticals.

General tips for getting you to 100 and beyond

Here are some more tips that don't fit into any of the other categories -

Get regular check-ups

This is one that many people are guilty of - they are so scared of the doctor's office that they avoid getting regular check-ups. Both my mother and grandmother died of problems that may have been treatable if they had sought help earlier. My mother knew something was wrong for a year before she was finally coerced into getting help. Remember this key fact - most cancers are curable if caught early. Cancer is not the death sentence it once was. However, once cancer has metastasized (spread) it becomes infinitely more difficult to treat, so you need to keep on top of things. If your doctor can identify and treat various problems early, your chances of beating them increase exponentially.

Order various tests

There are a range of tests that can be extremely helpful in illuminating existing or potential illnesses. The problem is that, unless your doctor has a specific concern, they won't order a test unless requested to.

The *c-reactive protein* (CRP) test is a great example. This test is used to detect inflammation in the body and is traditionally used to screen for heart disease where there is inflammation of the arteries suspected. A study that measured the CRP levels of 1100 men found that those with elevated CRP has triple the risk of heart disease and double the risk of stroke compared to those with normal or low levels. The CRP test is fantastic for identifying the very beginnings of heart disease, allowing you to put in place measures to prevent a possible heart attack from full-blown heart disease.

However there is also an association with elevated CRP and certain cancers. If you acknowledge that inflammation is one of the central factors in aging, then an accurate means to measure it is vital. When you ask for this test, make sure you ask for it in terms of your concern regarding heart disease.

At the same time, if you ask for a lipid panel to measure cholesterol, the key value to focus on is your triglycerides. Elevated triglycerides, which are associated with excess carbohydrate consumption, are increasingly being viewed as the best predictor of heart disease. While on the subject of lipid panel, try to get a particle-size test done. This measures the particle size of the lipoproteins because some particle sizes are benign, whereas others are harmful.

Some other tests to ask for including - vitamin D status, liver function, comprehensive metabolic panel, thyroid-stimulating hormone, complete blood cell count, fibrinogen, hemoglobin a1c, DHEA.

Some of these will be available and some you may need to visit a specialist laboratory.

Quantified self

Closely linked to the above topic of medical tests is the growing movement called quantified self. What this entails is measuring all aspects of your life empirically to enable to you to make positive changes or identify potential problems.

Probably the aspect of quantified self that you would be most familiar is pedometers that track the number of steps you take each day. This embodies one of the key concepts of quantified self - if you can measure something, you can improve it.

I own a *FitBit* tracker which I wear wherever I go. It tracks the number of steps, the distance, how many flights of stairs, calories burned and sleep quality. It tells me when I have been cooped up in my room writing for too long. I try to make it to 10,000 steps each day so when I find myself falling short, I go for a walk just to get to my target. This one little device has dramatically increased my activity levels. Unless I am in a skyscraper, I rarely ever take elevators any more, as I want to beat my record for most number of flights I have walked up in one day (currently 60 flights). I am a fan of FitBit but there are many different options so shop around if necessary.

Quantified self doesn't just refer to pedometers. It can refer to measuring various aspects of your body (waist size, weight etc.) and tracking the effects of certain activities. The central concept is that you can't improve what you can't measure. People can go years without weighing themselves or measuring their waistline then one day they hop on the scales and see a horrific number staring back at them. If you regularly track things like this, you have more opportunity to nip problems in the bud. Just don't go overboard. Remember, weight fluctuates wildly over a 24 or eve 48 hour period so don't keep weighing yourself each day. Once a week is enough - and make sure it's done at the same time each day.

Similarly, with a good quality blood pressure machine, if you take regular readings you will be able to identify and deal with any hypertension-related problems. Remember, hypertension (high blood pressure) is a silent killer. A good quality blood pressure machine could be the difference between life and death – literally.

Meditate regularly

Meditation has a range of longevity-enhancing effects, but the key benefit is secondary. Meditation is one of the best ways to combat chronic stress, which, as we know from earlier, is a huge driver of early death. Meditation leads to a range of physiological effects that reduce levels of stress, anxiety and depression.

Meditation is such a powerful anti-stress technique, that a whole new branch of psychotherapy, called *mindfulness-based stress reduction* (MBSR) has emerged as a popular way to fight stress and mood disorders. A 2003 meta-analysis found the MBSR was helpful not just for these obvious stress-related problems, but also for other conditions such as fibromyalgia, heart disease and certain other pain-related conditions.

Recent research into the effects of meditation on the brain, using fMRI and similar brain-scanning techniques, has thrown up some amazing results. One of the pioneers of this has been Professor Richard Davidson, director of the Laboratory for Affective Neuroscience at the University of Wisconsin, who has worked with the Dalai Lama to measure the brains of long term meditators. Among other things, Professor Davidson found that Tibetan lamas who had brains that were unlike any he had previously measured. When you think happy thoughts, certain parts of your brain (such as the left prefrontal cortex) light up. When you think negative or fearful thoughts, other parts light up (such as the right prefrontal cortex and the amygdala). Professor Davidson found a correlation between the number of hours someone meditates and the level of, what could subjectively be called "happiness".

The good news is that, while beginner meditators didn't have the extreme level of positive emotion in their brain after meditating, there were definite positive changes. These benefits of meditation slowly accrue over the long term.

Meditation also has direct effects on cellular aging. In particular, long term meditation is associated with higher levels of the important hormone DHEA, which usually decreases gradually as you age. Lower levels of DHEA (which is sometimes referred to as the "youth hormone") have been implicated in a range of conditions such as heart disease, diabetes and cancer. DHEA is considered so important, that many people have experimented with controversial DHEA supplementation. DHEA supplements are available in the US, but are still banned in most countries. My own personal philosophy is that I avoid any of these direct hormonal treatments such as DHEA or human growth hormone, as the research isn't yet conclusive regarding the risk/benefit ratio. The only hormone I supplement with is vitamin D (yes, it's a hormone and not actually a vitamin – fun fact!).

While meditation is now a mainstream, proven technique for stress reduction, there is still a huge amount of ignorance that prevents people from benefiting. Here are a couple of the main ones -

Meditation is against my religion - When it is boiled down to its purest essence, meditation is just a process of calming the mind and looking clearly at your own thought processes. Meditation (when used in a clinical setting) has become largely secular. There are virtually no widely-used meditation techniques that require you to compromise your beliefs to pray to any omnipresent being.

I tried meditating but I couldn't stop my thoughts - This is the most common roadblock that people erect. Meditating is not about stopping your thoughts. It is about calming down and then watching your thoughts. Trying to stop your thoughts is a sure-fire way to make yourself less relaxed, not more. Meditating is all about acceptance and letting go. Each time you find your train of thought wandering, just bring your attention back to the object of meditation (such as your breath) gently and start again.

Keep your core temperature down

OK, even I will admit this one is a bit whacky, but it is interesting enough that I wanted to include it.

Scientists have been experimenting with certain animals and have found that animals kept cooler tend to live longer. The theory is that the cooler temperatures slow down the rate of various metabolic processes and chemical reactions, theoretically slowing the aging process. For example, one study showed that by decreasing the core temperature of mice by 0.9 degrees Fahrenheit, researchers were able to extend the lifespan of mice by 20%.

The closest we have to replicating this in a practical manner in humans is through the consumption of *wasabi* – the hot horseradish used in Japanese sushi!

This is probably one for you to file away under "Useless Information", however I thought it was an interesting concept. My main problem is firstly that it doesn't seem to match up with the *Blue Zones*, which are mostly quite warm. I admit however that there could be a confounding factor – maybe the Blue Zone populations would live even longer if they pulled up sticks and moved to Greenland. My second problem is – even if this were verified, reducing your core temperature on a regular basis would be rather impractical. Short of building your own cool room or taking ice baths, it is fairly difficult to reduce you core temperature on a regular basis by any meaningful degree. One possible avenue is a drug that works similar to acetaminophen but without the glutathione-depleting aspects. As you may remember from last time you were sick and had a fever, acetaminophen can reduce body temperature a little.

If I can think of a single practical suggestion for reducing your average core body temperature it would be to switch some of your exercise focus to swimming. This could potentially kill two birds with one stone if you are also trying to manage your weight. The reduction in core temperature that accompanies swimming in cold water has been shown to dramatically increase your metabolic rate as your body works hard to bring your temperature back up to homeostasis. This is apparently the reason why Olympic swimmer Michael Phelps was able to consume such a huge number of calories each day and not gain weight. It was calculated that his energy consumption far outweighed his energy output from swimming, with the thermogenic effect of cold water the primary explanation.

Live a life of purpose

One of the great ironies of life is that many people spend their whole life working to that they can enjoy a comfortable retirement. They then reach this milestone and, lacking purpose, direction and structure to their day, they inexplicably die. For many years this has been a puzzling phenomenon. People retire and think that they will be able to just enjoy laying around all day reading the newspaper. Unfortunately for most people, our mind doesn't work that way. It needs purpose and direction to sustain it. Sometimes it almost seems as if your body takes retirement as a sign that its job here on Earth is done and it can now promptly expire.

For example a 2009 study of around 1200 elderly subjects found that those with a sense of purpose in life were half as likely to die in the five year study period as those without a sense of purpose. Half! That is an amazing figure. The study concluded *"Greater purpose in life is associated with a reduced risk of all-cause mortality among community-dwelling older persons"*

A sense of purpose is also believe to be a unifying factor in the Blue Zones which contributes to the greater life expectancy seen in these areas.

However the benefits are not just limited to the elderly. If we can just revisit stress, anxiety and depression for a moment, we will see that certain events or situation are not inherently bad – it is just that they are perceived to be negative by our own minds. If you are in a job that is incredibly demanding, depending on how you view your job, you will have a vastly different reaction on a cellular level.

Busyness does not equal stress. If you are doing what you love and you feel charged with purpose, you won't suffer the same biological consequences as someone trapped in a stressful, dead-end job.

Do what you can to give yourself a sense of purpose. Either change your situation or change how you view your situation.

Looking younger through appropriate skin care

I was initially planning to avoid mentioning skin care in this book because having "glowing" skin is not going to help you reach 100. However I have since taken some time to think about it and have changed my mind. The reason for this is that for many people, having younger looking skin makes them happy. They know that most of the invented, science-y sounding ingredients in their $100 jar of cream is not going to miraculously make them look 20 years younger. They know it is mostly marketing and placebo effect. But they don't care – because it makes them happy. The act of buying the latest cream advertised in Vanity Fair is enjoyable. The act of putting it on their skin is enjoyable. For many, this whole routine is like their own person Japanese tea ceremony.

Furthermore, I have realized that many people will be reading this book as part of a nascent personal makeover project. For these people, as well as feeling better they want to look better. And looking better makes them feel better.

Fortunately, there is one key fact that makes this a very easy section for me to write – Doing everything else in this book will be the single greatest thing they can do to achieve younger looking skin. Getting enough sleep and adopting a diet rich in omega 3 and antioxidants will do far more than most expensive skin care cream out there.

The good news also is that there are a few ingredients out there that actually work.

Firstly, we need to acknowledge that there are two types of skin aging – intrinsic and extrinsic. Intrinsic aging happens regardless of whether we look after our skin. As each year passes, there are changes to collagen and elastin fibers that eventually result in wrinkles and other signs of aging. Extrinsic aging refers to the environmental factors that accelerate the aging process of your skin. Fortunately there are things you can do to mitigate this process.

The beauty (pardon the pun) of anti-aging skin care is that all the concepts that apply to the rest of your body also apply to the skin. A large amount of the damage your skin sustains is caused by free radicals and advanced glycation end-products (AGEs). Remember the protein cross-linking I mentioned earlier that AGEs involve? That process is one of the reasons why prematurely aged skin looks more brittle and has less elasticity. So by following all the recommendations in this book regarding AGEs and antioxidants, you have already ticked a large box in terms of keeping your skin from aging prematurely.

However the number one premature ager of skin is UVA and UVB exposure from sunlight. This is where things get tricky because I believe that, as a society, we have developed the habit of avoiding sunlight due to perceived skin cancer risk, at the expense of our vitamin D status. And here is where it complicates further – one of the main processes of renewal that occurs in your skin – the production of keratinocytes – is controlled to a certain extent by vitamin D. Not complicated enough yet? Well, how about the fact that vitamin D itself has been shown to demonstrate photo-protective benefits for the skin? No problem, just put on sunscreen before you go outside so you get the vitamin D but without the skin-aging effects. Sorry – sunscreen blocks the absorption of ultraviolet light needed to trigger vitamin D production.

So, let's get this straight – You need vitamin D for a range of skin renewal and skin protection processes. You can't put on sunscreen or else you won't produce any vitamin D. So, logically you need to expose yourself to damaging ultraviolet light to get the anti-aging benefits of vitamin D. It's enough to give anyone a headache.

There are two ways to deal with this.

Firstly, carefully control both your exposure to sunlight and the areas of your body that are exposed. If you keep exposure to under twenty minutes or so, you are unlikely to suffer any real photo-damage. If you are concerned about premature aging to the skin on aesthetically important parts of your body (face, hands, neck etc.), try to get exposure to parts of your body that are not typically exposed. Here is something I experimented with in the name of this book. We have a sun lounge in our backyard. Once a day I laid down on the lounge, took my shirt off, covered my face and stayed there for around fifteen minutes or so. Theoretically, with whiter skin on the parts of your body that are not usually exposed, you should be able to produce vitamin D more effectively and require less time in the sun (*Note – this is an important point – the darker your skin, the less vitamin D you are able to produce from sunlight. This puts darker-skinned people who move to colder locations at greater risk of vitamin D deficiency*). If your skin goes red, you have stayed out too long.

Secondly, many dermatologists are now recommending a greater focus on dietary and supplemental vitamin D support instead of sun exposure. They are recommending anywhere from 4000-10,000IU per day from supplements to replace a large proportion of sun exposure. This way you will be getting all the benefits of vitamin D without the photoaging. The only downside is that your body has better control over its own vitamin D status when you are absorbing it mainly from the sun. It is able to switch off the production of vitamin D when levels are adequate. There is no risk of toxicity from sun exposure, which is one of the downsides of taking supplements. However I should also point out that there is a growing chorus of experts who have said that, unless massive doses are being taken each day, your risk of vitamin D toxicity is low. If you stick to 10,000IU and under per day, there is little risk of toxicity. However, as I have mentioned previously, ensure you add vitamin K supplements to your regime if you are taking more than a few thousand IU per day of vitamin D.

I am no expert on individual anti-aging creams. In fact, the whole beauty industry gives me an uncomfortable feeling the way it has no qualms about blatantly lying about the effectiveness of their products. However, I have dug into some research journals to separate fact from fiction. Even this is no guarantee that you will be able to avoid questionable ethics. For example, I stumbled on a paper which appeared to show a particular cream having superior anti-aging effects when compared to placebo. My excitement dimmed somewhat when I noticed down the bottom that the research study had been commissioned by the retail chain with exclusive selling rights to this particular cream!

I will risk further alienating the cosmetics industry when I tell you that by far the most effective anti-aging cream available is not even a retail product. It is only available on prescription from your doctor or dermatologist. This substance is a vitamin A retinoid known as *tretinoin* (Retin-A). What is particularly frustrating for the cosmetics industry is that they are allowed to use tretinoin in their own products, but only at concentrations so weak that they are virtually ineffective. If you want to try tretinoin you will have to get it via your doctor or dermatologist. Tretinoin has been shown to –

- Prevent and treat wrinkles effectively (don't expect miracles however)

- Prevent and treat age spots

- Assist in building collagen levels, creating a "younger-looking appearance" (this one is slightly vague for my liking)

In terms of the ingredients to look for in commercially available products, you should look for –

Ingredients that treat and prevent oxidative damage – vitamin C, green tea, idebenone, vitamin e

Ingredients that trigger skin renewal (such as collagen production) – retinol (make sure you avoid anything with *pro-retinols* like *retinyl palmitate, retinyl acetate*, and *retinyl linoleate*)

Ingredients that fill out wrinkles (temporarily lessening their appearance) - Hyaluronic Acid

Ingredients that trigger skin-cell turnover, giving a temporarily younger appearance – AHA, salicylic acid (BHA)

However probably the most overlooked way to prevent wrinkles from appearing and to temporarily lessen their appearance is to keep your skin well hydrated. Some ingredients to look for in products for both your face and body are – sorbolene (the cheapest and the best in many cases!), products using oats or shea butter.

Conclusion

As you will probably agree, that is a potentially confusing array of methods for increasing longevity. It's a lot to take in.

Company CEOs often like to get "1 pagers" from their staff that enables them to get across the issues without having to dig deep into the background or possibly unnecessary detail. So, here is my version of a 1-pager that summarizes everything you need to know in terms of increasing life expectancy –

- Avoid or reduce sources of stress

- Get enough sleep

- Don't smoke or abuse drugs (legal or otherwise). Reduce or eliminate alcohol

- Get regular exercise including cardiovascular exercise and weight training. Also ensure you include stretching and mobility-type exercise such as yoga or Pilates.

- Compulsory supplements for virtually everyone – omega 3 fatty acids (via fish oil, krill oil or even the more recent calamari oil), vitamin D, curcumin, n-acetylcystein, alpha lipoic acid. Plus optional supplements for decreasing oxidative stress such as resveratrol – if your budget allows

- Make educated decisions regarding medication. Always consider the risk/benefit ratio. If a medication will help you live longer or reduce suffering, take it. If it causes more problems than it treats, ditch it and investigate alternatives.

- Get at least 20 minutes of sunshine on your exposed skin each day. Don't go overboard with avoiding the sun altogether due to perceived skin cancer risk. You are more likely to get cancer from avoiding the sun (and getting vitamin D deficient) than you are from 20 minutes a day of sun exposure.

- Maintain a sense of purpose. Have a reason for getting out of bed each day.

- Maintain a rich network of social connections with friends and family. Avoid spending extended periods alone. A bit of solitary introspection is healthy. Too much is considerably unhealthier.

- Keep your brain healthy with intellectually stimulating activities and optional use of nootropic supplements that modulate dopamine and acetylcholine.

- Move to a Paleo-style diet. This doesn't mean you have to go "full Paleo" and ban all dairy, grains and legumes. In my case, I still eat all of those things but in much less quantity than I used to. Don't be a fundamentalist. If wheat doesn't cause you any problems – fine – keep eating it. However remember that some problems don't occur immediately, like where some people will get an immediate stomach ache after consuming wheat. The chronic, low level inflammation that wheat causes for many will take longer to reveal itself.

- The more vegetables you eat (particularly leafy greens), the longer you will live. This is one of the undisputed aspects of diet. Everyone agrees this point, whether they are up on the latest science or whether they are those conservative old nutritionists who still recommend plenty of "whole grains". Eat more veges.

- Regarding animal protein, where possible, try to switch your focus from red meat and chicken to seafood-based options like fish, squid, oysters etc.

- Closely monitor all possible aspects of your health and get regular check-ups.

- Engage in risky behavior with a full understanding that you are reducing your life expectancy. Each single episode of risky behavior is like playing Russian roulette using a gun with a lot of empty chambers. As risk increases, the number of empty chambers decreases.

- Always wear a sunscreen on your face to prevent premature photoaging.

If you find all this overwhelming, you can apply Pareto's law and just focus on –

- The causes of mortality over which you have the greatest control, and;

- The most common causes of mortality

For example, if you reduce your chances of dying from either heart disease, stroke or cancer, you have dramatically increased your chances of living past 100.

I feel I also need to address what is outside of our control.

Firstly, we need to acknowledge the impact of genetic makeup. While we don't know the exact proportion of effect, reaching 100 involves genetics to a certain degree. However, with each new research study that comes out, we are increasingly seeing the focus switch to interventions which can overcome genetic shortcomings. Don't become fatalistic. Focus on what you can control to mitigate any additional risk you may have of dying from a particular cause.

Secondly we need to at least give the power of *chance* a cursory glance. Yes, you could follow everything in this guide, have the cellular age of someone twenty years younger, yet still be run over by a bus tomorrow. Without wishing to get to philosophical, yes, our lives are always hanging by a thin gossamer thread. It is actually healthy to realize this – which is why a lot of meditative focus in Buddhism is directed towards appreciating that your time is limited, so you'd better make the most of this precious human birth we have been granted. All I can say is yes, chance could take your life at any minute, but remember that risk is additive. If you add in the chances of accidental death on top of accelerated cellular aging, you have almost no chance of reaching old age whatsoever. Focus on what you can control.

Before I go, I want to stress that this book is a living document that will regularly be updated as new research emerges. If we stay on the topic of Buddhism for a moment, once the Dalai Lama was asked what he would do if science disproved any aspect of what Buddhists believe, he replied *"If scientific analysis were conclusively to demonstrate certain claims in Buddhism to be false, then we must accept the findings of science and abandon those claims."*

Likewise, if new information emerges that disproves what we now believe, I will update my position. As I have stressed many times before – don't be fundamentalist about anything. If the consensus on wheat changes, I will be the first to load up on delicious croissants. However, where I stand now, I clearly know that croissants (one of my favorite foods on the planet by the way – it's my guilty secret) and other bread products make me put on weight and I feel slightly ill after eating them.

If you think I have gotten the science wrong, made an error or something in this book has become out of date due to new research, please let me know – jamesleetheauthor@gmail.com.

Above all, educate yourself and don't be afraid to experiment. In business, the key to experimentation is survival. If a company wishes to try a new strategy, this new strategy should not jeopardize the company's survival. Likewise, healthy experimentation is fine – just be aware of the risk/benefit ratio.

James Lee

January 2014

PS – If you found this book useful and you think others may benefit from it, please consider leaving a review here on Amazon. I will be eternally grateful (OK, maybe not eternally, but for a few weeks at least)

PPS – If you enjoyed this book, please check out my Amazon author page which has all my other books and guides.

41755935R00069

Made in the USA
San Bernardino, CA
20 November 2016